NEUROSCIENCE RESEARCH PROGRESS

RESEARCH TRENDS IN BEHAVIOR AND EXECUTIVE FUNCTION

NEUROSCIENCE RESEARCH PROGRESS

Additional books in this series can be found on Nova's website under the Series tab.

Additional e-books in this series can be found on Nova's website under the e-book tab.

NEUROSCIENCE RESEARCH PROGRESS

RESEARCH TRENDS IN BEHAVIOR AND EXECUTIVE FUNCTION

MIAO-KUN SUN
EDITOR

NOVA BIOMEDICAL

New York

NOTICE TO THE READER

Library of Congress Cataloging-in-Publication Data

Library of Congress Control Number: 2016941696
ISBN: 978-1-63485-461-0

Published by Nova Science Publishers, Inc. † New York

CONTENTS

PREFACE

This book brings together interdisciplinary research in cognitive psychology, cognitive impairment and abnormalities, cognitive networks and neurofeedback, and neurophysiology. Covered are the latest developments, pinpointing directions for future research on cognitive sciences and theory. Essential reading for those working directly in the cognitive sciences or in related specialist areas, "Research Trends in Behavior and Executive Function" provides an instant overview of current thinking for both experts and newcomers to cognitive sciences

Chapter 1 - Executive functioning refers to higher level fluid cognitive abilities that account for individual differences in planning and problem-solving. As such, these cognitive processes impact many aspects of daily functioning. Research has shown that neurological disorders, such as Parkinson's disease, Huntington's disease, multiple sclerosis, HIV, spina bifida, and Alzheimer's disease commonly result in deficits in executive processes and these conditions are covered in this review. The authors examine current models of executive functioning and explore current measures of executive functioning used in clinical practice as well as measures that are frequently used in experimental cognitive research. Lastly, the relation of executive functioning to neurological disorders and their treatment are discussed.

Chapter 2 - Increasing translational evidence suggests that long-chain omega-3 (LC*n*-3) fatty acids, including eicosapentaenoic acid (EPA, 20:5*n*-3) and docosahexaenoic acid (DHA, 22:6*n*-3), play a critical role in brain development. DHA has anti-inflammatory, neurotrophic, and neuroprotective properties and accumulates in the brain during active periods of perinatal cortical expansion and functional connectivity. Rodent studies demonstrate that reductions in perinatal rat brain DHA accrual are associated with delays in neuronal migration and arborization, synaptic pathology, neurocognitive deficits, and elevated behavioral indices of aggression and depression. Non-human primates raised on an *n*-3 fatty acid deficient diet exhibit hyperactivity, impairments in visual attention, and functional connectivity deficits within cortical networks. Human preterm delivery is associated with early deficits in cortical DHA accrual, enduring reductions in cortical circuit connectivity, and increased risk for developing psychiatric disorders including unipolar depression, bipolar disorder, and schizophrenia. These psychiatric disorders commonly initially emerge during adolescence, a developmental period associated with rapid and dynamic changes cortical circuit maturation, and are associated with LC*n*-3 fatty acid deficits. This body of translational evidence suggests that deficits in LC*n*-3 fatty acids during perinatal development may contribute to impaired cortical circuit maturation and associated risk for psychiatric disorders. Developing a more comprehensive understanding of the requirement for LC*n*-3 fatty acids during normal human perinatal brain development could therefore have significant implications for informing optimal intake levels during critical periods of neurodevelopment.

Chapter 3 - Executive functions involve a series of cognitive, behavioral and affective-emotional components, which play an important role regulating and organizing one´s behavior in a wide range of situations, especially in those that require a creative and novel approach. The impact of these components is especially noticeable either on social, academic and clinical settings. This has led many authors to consider executive functions as a core aspect predicting social adaptation, as well as an important asset in the diagnosis and intervention in several childhood and adolescence disorders. This prominence given to executive functions suggests the need for reliable and valid assessment tools, and even more importantly, the need for an adequate body of information that helps researchers and professionals to successfully interpret results from empiric evidence. This chapter is aimed at addressing both aspects. Thus, the authors focus on analyzing the main features of the assessment tools available today and to what extent they are suitable for their application in clinical and educational settings, paying special attention to new perspectives and instruments. Finally, the authors outline some suggestions intended to improve election, application and interpretation of the results gathered in the evaluation process.

Chapter 4 - The relationship between stress and executive functioning is bidirectional and complex. This manuscript focuses on the relationship of stress and executive functioning with respect to both negative and positive outcomes. First, the authors highlight the negative impact of stress upon executive functioning. This is followed by a discussion of how executive dysfunction impacts the ability to recover from stress. The authors then move into a discussion of the positive impacts of stress upon executive functioning. Lastly, the authors discuss how the presence of intact executive functioning can positively impact the process of coping with stress.

Chapter 5 - In neuroimaging paradigms, reappraisal has received considerable attention as an effective emotion regulation strategy but most studies have instructed participants to 'reappraise' impersonal emotion-evoking stimuli as opposed to real-life events and have not given specific guidance regarding how to reappraise. Big picture reappraisal is a specific emotion regulation strategy that offers a way of managing distress aiming to promote acceptance and cognitive coping. Big picture reappraisal instructions resulted in activation in bilateral superior parietal lobe, associated with abstraction, as well as areas associated with cognitive control of emotion (orbital frontal cortex, medial prefrontal cortex, lobule VI cerebellum) when compared to distraction and rumination instructions.

Chapter 6 - Traumatic brain injury (TBI) is a major problem of public health around the world. TBI is a neurological disorder that results in temporary or permanent changes in motor, cognitive and behavioral areas. It is one of the most common kinds of brain injuries in childhood/adolescence, a period in which the prefrontal cortex is in a developing process. The aim of this article is to review the neuropsychological consequences of TBI in the prefrontal cortex, as well as the valid strategies to be adopted that might contribute to a shorter recovery time of the patients. The TBI in the prefrontal cortex does not necessarily involve motor or sensorial deficits. However, it may cause functional, decision making, and social and academic impairments. More than a half of these patients develop a psychiatric disorder with disinhibiting symptoms and inappropriate behavior. Motivational, emotional, attention, perceptive and cognitive functions are mediated by the connections between the prefrontal cortex and the motor areas, the limbic system, the reticular system and the posterior association cortex. Generally, patients with TBI will present cognitive deficits associated with executive functions, decision making, problem-solving skills, judgment, and impulse control. The consequences of brain injury depend on a variety of factors, such as: the type of brain injury, intensity of the damage, extension, localization, environmental factors, age in which the TBI occurs, premorbid intelligence/cognitive reserve, and stage of cognitive development. For example, dorsolateral lesions have been associated with perseverative behavior, lack of initiative, deficit in ability to sustain and shift attention between stimuli or concepts, problem solving and working memory ("cold" executive functions). It is commonly confused with unmotivated behavior. On the other hand, ventromedial injuries have been associated with conducts based on emotional and social variables, such as inability to respond appropriately to social cues, failure to obey conventional social rules, inhibitory deficits, impulsivity and impaired decision making ("hot" executive functions). Right after the brain injury, new mechanisms of repair and reorganization of the Central Nervous System (CNS) emerge for an indefinite time period, aiming to reduce and compensate the functional impairment associated with the problem. A new neuronal circuit in the neighbor areas of the brain is established to recover lost functions and consequently to help the accomplishment of activities. The process of restructuring the brain and strengthening the cognitive functions is called neural plasticity and it can improve the prognostic of the subject at any stage of development or adult life. In most patients, when the brain injury in the prefrontal cortex happens, special educational needs or changes in the educational environment are necessary. In the meantime, there are promising treatments with stimulant drugs, neuropsychological rehabilitation, and cognitive behavioral therapy strategies. Further studies on neuropsychological rehabilitation are required to define to what extent individuals affected by TBI may have a restoration of premorbid cognitive abilities by making use of these integrated techniques.

Chapter 7 - The cerebellum is increasingly recognized as a structure that regulates cognitive and emotional functioning in much the same way that it modulates motor activity. Reciprocal connections with prefrontal and temporoparietal association cortices facilitate cerebellar modulation of implicit learning and executive functions, while connections with paralimbic regions allow for cerebellar regulation of emotional responses. Furthermore, recent evidence indicates that the cerebellum is reciprocally connected with the basal ganglia, forming an interconnected subcortical network with an extensive influence on cortical processing. In this review, the authors first discuss the neuroanatomical basis of the cerebellum's role in implicit learning and executive functioning. Next, the authors examine evidence of cerebellar contributions to executive dysfunction in select neurological and psychiatric illnesses. The authors conclude with a brief discussion regarding potential treatments targeting the cerebellum.

In: Research Trends in Behavior …
Editor: Miao-Kun Sun
ISBN: 978-1-63485-461-0

Chapter 1

EXECUTIVE FUNCTIONING IN COMMON NEUROLOGIC CONDITIONS

Benjamin D. Hill*, Rachel Hoadley, Katherine F. Russ, Emily Corley and Joseph P. Pastuszak
Department of Psychology, University of South Alabama, Mobile, Alabama, US

ABSTRACT

Executive functioning refers to higher level fluid cognitive abilities that account for individual differences in planning and problem-solving. As such, these cognitive processes impact many aspects of daily functioning. Research has shown that neurological disorders, such as Parkinson's disease, Huntington's disease, multiple sclerosis, HIV, spina bifida, and Alzheimer's disease commonly result in deficits in executive processes and these conditions are covered in this review. We examine current models of executive functioning and explore current measures of executive functioning used in clinical practice as well as measures that are frequently used in experimental cognitive research. Lastly, the relation of executive functioning to neurological disorders and their treatment are discussed.

* Correspondence and requests for reprints: Benjamin D. Hill, Ph.D., UCOM 1032, Department of Psychology, University of South Alabama, Mobile, AL 36688; office phone 251-460-7081; bdhill@southalabama.edu.

Keywords: executive functioning, Parkinson's disease, Huntington's disease, multiple sclerosis, HIV, spina bifida, Alzheimer's disease

1. INTRODUCTION

Executive functioning (EF) has long been vital in understanding the social and cognitive implications of brain injury. For example, most introductory psychology courses discuss the case of the railroad worker Phineas Gage, who had a metal rod pierce and exit his skull, damaging his left prefrontal cortex and white matter. Despite Gage's injury, his health was described as "good," but he exhibited significant changes in personality with a marked increase in disinhibited and vulgar behaviors. Executive abilities such as planning, problem-solving, and reasoning skills were all also reported impaired in Mr. Gage and he was unable to return to his previous job as a supervisor or hold other meaningful employment (Damasio, Grabowski, Frank, Galaburda, and Damasio, 1994).

This case exemplified the significant relationship executive abilities have to our everyday functioning. From the moment we awaken to the time we go to sleep, we utilize these abilities. For example, taking a shower requires aspects of working memory ("I just washed my left shoulder so I don't need to do that again"), ordered planning ("shampoo before conditioner"), and inhibition ("my phone just rang, let it go to voicemail rather than answering it in the shower"). Due to our heavy reliance on executive functions in activities of daily living, people with neurologic conditions that affect executive abilities often requires assistance at least some minimal assistance from caregivers and loved ones in their lives.

This review will focus on executive functioning in medical populations. First, we will discuss a prominent theory of executive functioning, the development of executive skills, and the neuroanatomical substrates of executive functioning. Next, we will cover common assessment methods for measuring executive functions. We will also describe specific neurological disorders where executive dysfunction is common, including Parkinson's disease, Huntington's disease, multiple sclerosis (MS), human immunodeficiency virus (HIV), and spina bifida (SB). Lastly, we will elaborate on the impact of executive dysfunction on the individual diagnosed with these disorders.

2. Model of Executive Functioning

We believe one of the best supported current conceptualizations of executive functioning is Miyake and Friedman's (2000) model. This model proposes three underlying components which account for individual differences in executive functions: mental set shifting ("shifting"), information updating and monitoring ("updating"), and the inhibition of dominant or prepotent responses. According to this model of executive functioning, these components are latent variables which influence performance on all tasks which index executive abilities.

2.1 Shifting

Shifting is the ability to shift one's attention back and forth between multiple tasks, operations, or mental sets. Executive shifting can be found in many behaviors we do in everyday life, such as driving where there are multiple gauges that require routine monitoring while we also allocate attention to the road and conversations in the car. Shifting may also account for more abstract tasks or cognitive ability such as summation. This ability has also been named "task switching" or "attention switching" by other authors (Miyake, Friedman, Emerson, Witzki, and Howerter, 2000). Monsell (2003) described every day activities such as reading while eating breakfast as behavioral examples of shifting. It is generally believed that different neural networks mediate the shifting of visual attention versus more executive-oriented shifts (Raichle, 1994).

2.2 Updating

Updating refers to the act of monitoring and encoding new information to replace older and potentially outdated information. Miyake and colleagues (2000) stated that updating is not simply passively storing recent information over old information, but an active manipulation of incoming information. This active adaptation of information is vastly different from merely storing both old and new information separately. Passive storage activates the premotor areas of the frontal cortex and parietal regions whereas updating is associated with the dorsolateral prefrontal cortex, an area associated with working memory (Jonides et al., 1997). For example, you are updating while reading this right now as new information enters working memory and replaces the concepts you have previously read.

2.3 Inhibition

The last component of Miyake and Friedman's (2000) executive functioning model is the ability to deliberately inhibit dominant, prepotent, or automatic responses. Inhibition is extremely important in everyday life. It is the cognitive ability that keeps you from looking at the attractive individual who just walked into the room when you are sitting beside your significant other (a skill sometimes learned through painful experience). It is the executive ability that keeps you from cursing when you stump your toe in front of your child. Clinically, impairment in the inhibition component of executive functioning is most likely to prevent patients from returning to their previous employment or resume normal social interactions. The children's game "Simon says" is difficult for young children precisely because inhibitory skills are still developing in childhood.

There is considerable research support for Miyake and Friedman (2000) model of executive functions but the original three factor model was demonstrated largely in young adults. Fisk and Sharp (2004) conducted a factor analysis using an age diverse sample who completed measures designed to tap into the constructs of shifting, updating, and inhibition. They found four factors rather than the three components described by Miyake and Friedman. The last factor was the efficiency of access to long-term memory (unrelated to aging) and was conceptualized to be a different form of processing speed. Similarly, Adrover-Roig, Sese, Barcelo, and Palmer (2012) replicated this same four factor structure of executive functioning. Their sample was approximately the same size as Fisk and Sharp (2004) but with an older population. It is possible that when considering older populations, that processing speed related to memory retrieval has a large influence on the efficiency and accuracy of executive functions than is found in younger individuals.

3. Functional Neuroanatomy of Executive Functioning

Executive functions have historically been conceptualized as an ability of the prefrontal cortex (PFC). The PFC is the region of the brain located anterior to the motor and premotor cortices and the supplementary motor area. The left PFC is associated with the initiation of responses and processing verbal, concrete, or detail-oriented information. The right PFC is associated more with inhibition of responses (Suchy, 2009).

The PFC can be subdivided into three regions. Schon, Ross, Hasselmo, and Stem (2013) found that the first region, the dorsolateral prefrontal cortex (DLPFC), is related to encoding and updating working memory. This same region has also been associated with planning (Kaller, Rahm, Spreer, Weiller, and Unterrainer, 2011). More specifically, a functional magnetic resonance imaging (fMRI) study by these researchers described the left DLPFC as performing planning tasks like goal hierarchies or the sequencing of plans to reach a goal. They found that the right DLPFC is more focused on search depth or the cognitive task of generating steps toward the goals. Further, so-called "cold" or "cool" executive functions that relate to pure attentional allocation are more associated with the DLPFC than other regions (Takeuchi et al., 2013). Cold executive functions include working memory, planning, and problem solving. "Hot" executive functions are associated with mediating social interactions and affect.

Bledsoe, Semrud-Clikeman, and Plizska (2013) determined that the second region, the supero-medial prefrontal cortex (SMPFC), which includes the anterior cingulate cortex (ACC), is related to inhibition and executive control. Suchy (2009) added motivation to this list of functions, as well as the encoding or labeling of stimuli and experiences as positive or negative. Further, Gasquoine (2013) stated that a number of studies have found the ACC to be related to psychopathology, including obsessive-compulsive disorder, major depressive disorder, substance abuse disorders, as well as Attention-Deficit/Hyperactivity Disorder (ADHD; Bledsoe Semrud-Clikeman, and Plizska, 2013). The bulk of evidence suggests that the ACC is involved with sustained attention and response selection. In other words, the ability to maintain attention on the task at hand and respond to the correct stimuli, such as driving through congested traffic and responding to other drivers rather than a ringing cell phone, is an executive task.

The third region of the PFC is the ventral prefrontal cortex (VPFC), which can be divided into the orbitofrontal prefrontal cortex (OFC) and the ventromedial prefrontal cortex (vmPFC). The OFC is associated with hot executive functioning such as affective decision-making (Zelazo and Carlson, 2012) and processing social information. For example, Ross, LoPresti, Schon and Stern (2013) found that when participants attempted to identify a face they just recently saw or saw after an extended period of time, the OFC worked in conjunction with the hippocampus in this working memory task. Further, Willis, Palermo, McGrillen, and Miler (2014) found that compared to normal controls those who have sustained damage to the OFC have a substantially impaired ability to recognize facial expressions. On the other hand, the vmPFC is related to risk assessment in planning (Rogalsky, Vidal, Li, and Damasio, 2012).

Despite the fact that executive functions are strongly associated with the frontal cortices, Suchy (2009) has emphasized that other areas of the brain contribute to executive abilities. However, the frontal lobes have deep, rich connections to other parts of the brain, mainly through the striatum to parietal cortices. Thus, the frontal lobes act as a processing center as well as a highway to other cortical substrates involved in executive functions. For example, working memory tasks activate the dorsolateral prefrontal cortex in conjunction with the parietal lobes and sometimes the hippocampus. Another example would be that attentional switching also utilizes the basal ganglia and the thalamus in conjunction with the medial and ventral PFC.

It may be that individual differences result from variations in structure or connectivity to these structures. Additionally, there may be differences in cortical thickness. Burzynska and colleagues (2012) administered the Wisconsin Card Sort Task (WCST), which is a common neuropsychological test of attention, updating, and inhibition while participants were undergoing fMRI imaging. While DLPFC thickness was most important for WCST performance, it was also associated with the right DLPFC, right ventrolateral PFC, the superior parietal cortex (for working memory), and the ACC. They found that while decreases in cortical thickness were sometimes related to executive dysfunction, variations in cortical thickness between individuals was often unrelated to executive functioning performance. Ruscheweyh and colleagues (2013) conducted a similar study with different measures of switching, updating, and inhibition. They found that the updating task was related to DLPFC cortical thickness, switching was related to the DLPFC and ventrolateral prefrontal cortical thickness, and inhibition was associated with left DLPFC and ACC cortical thickness.

4. Development of Executive Functions

Executive functioning is known to be sensitive to aging. It is one of the last cognitive abilities to mature and one of the earliest to be affected by normal aging in older adults (Best, Miller, and Jones, 2009). The PFC develops similarly to other cortical areas and requires neuronal proliferation, new synapse formation, myelination of axons, pruning, and apoptosis, though at a much slower rate. Basic motor and sensory functions develop much sooner than executive abilities illustrating the hierarchical nature of executive functions that require other lower level abilities to build upon (Best, Miller, and Jones, 2009). For example, children typically develop motor skills like crawling faster than they develop language skills like talking with the ability to plan or engage in strategic game play coming even later.

According to a review by Best, Miller, and Jones (2009), executive functions begin to noticeably emerge at approximately three years of age. This initiation of growth appears to be related to the development of the PFC. Shifting abilities have been documented to emerge around three to four years of age and continues to develop until mid-adolescence. As for working memory, there is a linear progression from ages four to fifteen years. However, there is no real change in improvement in ages nine to twenty years in working memory of facial recognition. Inhibition is reported to begin early in development, but has a rapid growth period between five and eight years of age. Lastly, planning typically develops in late childhood and continues into late adolescence. These developmental trajectories depend upon normal early development and may not apply in atypical cases. For example, premature children (less than thirty weeks of gestation) frequently have later deficits in executive functioning (Aarnoudse-Moens, Weisglas-Kuperus, Duivenvoorden, Oosterlaan, and van Goudoever, 2012). These deficits appear to be due to diffuse white matter abnormalities and differences in frontal cortical thickness. Conversely, children who have higher postnatal growth are reported to have less executive dysfunction.

There is evidence that environmental as well as biological factors may influence the development of executive functions. Lawson, Duda, Avants, Wu, and Farah (2013) found greater cortical thickness in children of parents who had parents with higher educational attainment. This was postulated to be due either to inherited parental genetics related to executive functioning or possibly to parents with more education investing more in their child's cognitive development. In addition to parental education, parenting quality appears to moderate executive development. Blair, Raver, and Berry (2014) compared children at 36 and 60 months of age on measure of executive functioning and parenting quality. Parental quality predicted change in executive functioning over time, but executive functioning also predicted parental quality. That is, children who showed greater executive abilities were more likely to receive better parenting in the form of maternal scaffolding, sensitivity, and support for autonomy, which mirrors leading developmental theories.

While studies in adults have found three or four factor models for executive functioning (Miyake and Friedman, 2000; Adrover-Roig et al., 2012; Fisk and Sharp, 2004), the typical shifting, updating, and inhibition structure has not been consistently replicated in children suggesting a strong developmental aspect to the Miyake and Friedman model. An example is a study where van der Ven, Kroesbergen, Boom, and Leseman (2013) conducted a factor analysis of executive functioning measures in 6-year-olds. They were unable to replicate a factor structure similar to Miyake et al. (2000), and instead found that measure of inhibition cross loaded on switching, updating, and two separate processing speed factors. Therefore, it appears the cognitive architecture of executive functioning changes over time and suggests that the executive components are initially combined and begin to separate early on, becoming updating, shifting, and inhibiting in young adulthood with processing speed becoming more integral to executive abilities as we age.

5. Measuring Executive Functioning

Many types of measurement have been suggested in studying executive functioning. Some common methods of measurement have included lesion mapping, brain imaging, behavioral self- and other-reports, cognitive computerized tasks, and clinician-administered tests. All of these methods of measurement can be categorized two ways: experimental (cognitive) measures or clinical (applied) measures. Both types of measures are used in research and the clinical measures have traditionally begun as experimental tasks that demonstrated diagnostic utility and were translated into clinical use. Currently, many measures are used both clinically and experimentally.

In researching the experimental measurement of executive functioning, the majority of the literature describes using clinical measures in an experimental setting (Morgan and Lilienfeld, 2000; Schnitzspahn, Stahl, Zeintl, and Kaller, 2012; Tannock, 1998). This is logical considering that measures must be validated experimentally before utilized clinically. That said, a number of cognitive psychologists have measured executive functioning, specifically updating, inhibition, and task switching. Often, these cognitive paradigms can evolve quicker than clinical tests that have to be validated and normed before use with patients. This process can take several years, which results in the experimental measures often being years ahead of the clinical assessments from a theoretical and current best conceptualization standpoint. Consistent with Miyake and Friedman's model of executive functioning, measures used to analyze task shifting, inhibition, and updating will be the functions most pertinent to our discussion.

6. Measuring Task Shifting

At the most basic level, this involves requiring a participant to follow one set or directive, and have that person switch to a different task or different set of directions. Experimentally, Sylvester and colleagues (2003) used functional brain imaging to assess task switching. More behaviorally, Salthouse et al. (1998) have used two novel experimental tasks, the digit-digit task and digit-symbol task, to evaluate task switching. In the digit-digit task, both items in the pair are digits. In the digit-symbol task, one item is a number and the other a symbol. The participant must consult a code in order to determine if their numerical values are equivalent. Then, the participant must indicate whether or not they are identical. The main limitation was that the operations involved in the digit-symbol task were more cognitive in nature and, thus, not a perfect comparison to the digit-digit task. A second experimental way executive switching has been evaluated is by measuring the efficiency of switching. This involves measuring the cost of switching between sets in terms of time and accuracy. This most common clinical measure to adopt this paradigm is the venerable Trail Making Test (TMT), part B. This test involves alternating between numbers (1-25) and letters of the alphabet putting both in the correct order. TMT part B requires the individual both to maintain a response set and simultaneously switch between sets.

7. Measuring Updating

Updating is a more direct way to describe the function served by working memory: maintaining old information while integrating new information simultaneously. The classic lag task, better known as the n-back task, is an excellent example of an updating task as the individual has to keep a running tally of presented items in order to give the correct answer. Experimentally, Schnitzspahn and colleagues (2013) have used the computerized keep-track task and the letter-memory task to measure updating. The keep-track task involved five trials mixed with a list of fifteen words from one of six semantic categories. The participants tried to remember the last exemplar from each semantic cluster. The letter-memory task involved another list, which consisted only of letters. From each trial, the participant was to recall the last three letters.

Validated clinical measures of updating include the Sentence Span, Digit Span Backward, and the Self-Ordered Pointing tasks (Willcutt, Doyle, Nigg, Faraone, and Pennington, 2005). Sentence Span refers to a participant reproducing each word after all sentences are completely read. Digit Span Backward requires that the participant repeats the list of digits spoken but in reverse order. Self-ordered pointing demands that the participant select a novel design on each presented card.

8. Measuring Inhibition

Generally, task that measure inhibition require a participant to inhibit a dominant response. A classic example is the many variations of the Go-No Go paradigm that have been utilized across disciplines and even species to assess executive functioning. Experimentally, the Stop-Signal Reaction Time task has been used to evaluate a person's ability to inhibit (Willcutt, Doyle, Nigg, Faraone, and Pennington, 2005). Another cognitive measure of inhibition involves neuroanatomical findings to try to establish inhibitory functioning (Castellanos et. al, 2006). Likewise, Aron, Robbins, and Poldrack (2004) detected that neuroimaging indicated several different prefrontal cortex foci for active inhibition functions. Conversely, they found that human lesion mapping showed that it was isolated to the right inferior frontal cortex. The most common task used to assess inhibition in ADHD literature (Tannock, 1998) is the Continuous Performance Test (CPT). There are at least two types of CPT methodologies, one that requires to person to only respond to a specific stimulus and ignore all other stimuli and another that requires the person to respond to all stimuli expect for a specific stimulus. The latter method is generally more sensitive to inhibitory deficits in ADHD. Perhaps the oldest test to be used experimentally and clinically to assess inhibition is the

Stroop paradigm which dates back to at least 1935. In the Stroop task, the person is shown the name of a color (such as “blue”) that is printed in a color of ink that is inconsistent with the word (e.g., "blue" in yellow ink). The Stroop task involves having the person read the word on the first trial to activate this overlearned, prepotent response. Next, the person is asked to state the color that the word is printed in rather than reading the word. This requires the person to inhibit the automatic process of reading the word.

Many traditional clinical tests of executive functioning measure aspects of all three executive components. For example, the Wisconsin Card Sorting Test (WCST) requires both switching from a previously learned response pattern and inhibition of the previously correct response set. The Controlled Oral Word Association Test (COWAT), another relatively common clinical measure used to assess language processing associated with executive functioning, requires updating of previously said words, shifting to new phonemic categories, and inhibition of previously said word to maximize performance.

9. Neuropsychological Measurement of Executive Functioning

Experimental psychological measures frequently influence the development of clinical tests. An area of clinical psychology that strives to combine the cognitive literature with application is neuropsychology, often resulting in a blurring of the line between experimental and clinical cognitive measures. Neuropsychologists specialize in the assessment and evaluation of brain-behavior relationships and have particularly contributed to the development of measures to examine executive functioning.

Executive functioning as a global construct has been of particular importance to clinicians. In 2000, Morgan and Lilienfeld conducted a meta-analytic review of hyperactive behavior and neuropsychological measures of executive function. They described the difficulty in discerning executive dysfunction via existing measures. In their meta-analysis, they reviewed a variety of validated measures including, the perseverative error score on the Wisconsin Card Sorting Test (WCST), verbal fluency tests such as the COWAT, the Category Test of the Halstead-Reitan Neuropsychological Battery (HRNB), the Qualitative (Q) score on the Porteus Mazes Test, the Stroop Test, and TMT part B. Their inclusion criteria were that each of the tests had to incorporate one of the domains of executive functioning and had been shown to differentiate patients with and without focal frontal lobe lesions. Overall, their findings indicated that these tests were valid measures of executive functioning.

10. Comparisons of Types of Measurement

10.1 Self-report vs. Neuropsychological Assessment

Anderson examined a self-report measure of executive functioning, the Behavior Rating Inventory of Executive Function (BRIEF; 2002). The BRIEF is an 86-item questionnaire that an adult patient or parent of a patient confirms or denies global manifestations of executive functioning. Results suggested that that the BRIEF score was not significantly related to cognitive measures of executive functioning (Anderson, 2002).

10.2 Cognitive vs. Clinical Assessments

Though the lines between clinical and experimental measures have been blurred at times, comparing clinical and cognitive constructs of executive functioning is important for the field of neuropsychology. It is often unclear how well the cognitive neuroscience literature translates to the clinical domain as there is a relative paucity of studies comparing experimental measures of executive functioning to traditional clinical measures. This type of direct comparison is needed to address whether or not different tasks actually tap into the same construct.

Shelton, Elliott, Hill, Calamia, and Gouvier (2011) examined precisely this grey area using a broad battery of clinical and experimental tests of executive abilities with a focus on working memory. They found that experimental measures such as Operation Span (which entails solving basic math problems while also remembering a string of letters), Listening Span (which required the participant to recall the last word from a number of sentences in order), and the Modified Lag Task (a verbal n-back task) were generally the best indicators of fluid cognitive abilities, though the clinical measures did index the same construct as the experimental measures. The clinical measures they compared to these experimental measures were Digit

Span, Arithmetic, and Letter Number Sequencing from the Wechsler Adult Intelligence Scale, Third Edition (WAIS-III). They also found that WAIS-III subtests Block Design, not usually considered a measure of executive ability, was more strongly related to criterion fluid intelligence constructs than subtests such as Matrix Reasoning. Additionally, Bull and Scerif (2001) found overall strong correlations between cognitive and clinical test they studied. Namely, interference on the Stroop task was associated with perseverative errors on the WCST. Similarly, Salthouse, Atkinson, and Berish (2003) examined various executive functioning measures and found them to be highly related. In some of their models, these constructs exhibited both convergent and divergent validity.

11. Neurological Disorders

So far we have discussed executive functioning and the impact this domain has on cognitive processes. Executive functioning contributes significantly to successful cognitive processing and overall psychological functioning. In those with neurological disorders, deficits in executive functioning lead to noticeable impairments and negatively affect the individual's quality of life. To demonstrate how deficits with executive functioning manifest in individuals with neurological disorders, we will be discussing seven different neurological disorders.

11.1 Parkinson's Disease

First described in 1817 by James Parkinson's, Parkinson's disease (PD) represents one of the most common neurological disorders today, second only to Alzheimer's Disease (Carlson, Eldreth, Chuang, and Eaton, 2012). Currently, PD is diagnosed at a rate of 40,000 cases in the United States annually (Weintraub, Comella, and Horn, 2008). Typically the disease has a 1.5 to 2 times higher prevalence rate in men compared to women. Additionally, the disease is known to develop an average 2.1 years later in women than in men. Differences in symptomology also occur between genders. For instance, more women (67%) present with a Parkinsonian tremor compared to men (48%; Haaxma et al., 2007). Even though the literature on

PD has expanded, researching the disorder is problematic due to difficulty establishing the diagnosis.

Van Den Eeden and colleagues (2002) noted that the low base rate of PD (1-3% of the population depending on age) and delayed symptom presentation complicated diagnosis. They evaluated a sample of 588 patients with PD in order to decipher age, race and gender trends for the disorder. They found that 61% of their sample was male, reflecting previous findings suggesting a higher ratio in men than women. Similarly, the majority of patients fell between the ages of 60-69 (N=154) and 70-79 (N= 259). This is also consistent with previous findings suggesting a prevalence rate of PD affecting 1-3% of the population above 65 years (Dirnberger and Jahanshahi, 2013; de Rijk et al., 2000).

11.1.1. Cognitive Impairments

Cognitive impairments can be found in approximately 18-36% of patients (Dirnberger and Jahanshahi. 2013; Aarsland et al., 2009; Foltynie, Brayne, Robbins and Barker, 2004). While attention and language abilities seem to remain mostly intact, individuals with PD are bradyphrenic, which involves difficulties with processing speed of information (Dauer and Przedborski, 2003). For example, individuals with PD will often take longer to respond to a question than their healthy counterparts. Other neuropsychological impairments may be reported in the domains of memory, visuospatial skills, inhibitory control, and processing speed (Muslimovic, 2005).

Executive dysfunction is believed to be the most defined cognitive impairment, affecting roughly 30% of PD patients (Parker, Lamichhane, Caetano, and Narayanan, 2013; Williams-Gray et al., 2009; Aarsland and Kurz, 2010; Dirnberger and Jahanshahi, 2013; Calabresi et al., 2006). Due to the depletion of dopaminergic neurons, individuals with Parkinson's have difficulties inhibiting automated responses and retrieving previously learned information from memory, planning as well as with effortful processing, action selection, problem solving, verbal fluency, cognitive flexibility, and generating new rules and response sets (Calabresi et al., 2006; Muslimovic et al., 2005; Wylie et al., 2010; Kudlicka, Clare, and Hindle, 2013).

11.1.2. Shifting deficits

Individuals with PD are also impaired on measures of dual-task performance (Dirberger and Jahanshahi, 2013; Brown and Marsden, 1998). Dual task-performance is the concurrent performance of two tasks and is related to shifting. For example, Brown and Marsden (1998) found that those with PD demonstrated difficulty with completing a Stroop task while intermittingly completing a secondary task such as random letter generation. Results suggested significant impairment on the Stroop task relative to healthy controls.

Achieving success on dual-task performance involves switching attention. Studies have shown that those with PD have difficulties with attention such as shifting attention and with dual-task performance. Cools and colleagues (2001) evaluated difficulties with set shifting by having individuals switch between letter and naming tasks every second trial. Their findings indicated that individuals with PD showed significant difficulties with tasks of set shifting. This was present during the earliest stages of the disease. Further emphasizing the finding, those with PD showed impairment on set shifting, but impairment only occurred only when they had to inhibit competing information.

11.1.3. Updating deficits

Updating or working memory refers to the abstract reasoning that allows a person to multi-task, such as recalling numbers while also being able to rank order those numbers. Another way to consider it is as the ability to update and integrate new information into previously existing schemas. Deficits in working memory have been noted in PD when compared to normal updating capacities, particularly in the manipulation of new information (Gilbert, Belleville, Bherer, and Choinard, 2005). These discrepancies were significantly greater than even the impairments due to motor and psychomotor dysfunction.

11.1.4. Inhibition deficits

In healthy individuals, inhibition is the ability to suppress a response or action that may be inappropriate, or the ability to ignore an outside stimulus to maintain attention. In those with PD, inhibition is impaired (Cooper, Sagar, Tidswell, and Jordan, 1994; Dinberger and Jahanshahi, 2013). More recently, Favre and colleagues (2013) explored proactive inhibition in PD. Proactive inhibition is when different associations correlate with one another. In other words, it is the tendency for earlier learned information to interfere with the ability to retain new information and it is impaired in those with PD.

11.1.5 Impact

Many of the cognitive deficits discussed so far correlate with motor symptoms of the disease. For instance, one study found that executive dysfunction in those with PD relates to symptoms of postural instability (Nocera et al., 2010). Postural instability refers to unstable balance and gait within the individual which increases their likelihood of falling. Postural instability in PD is associated with poorer performance on tests of attention and executive functioning (Nocera et al., 2010). Additionally, Allcock and colleagues (2009) found that patients with severe gait difficulties and frequent falls performed more poorly on tests of attention relative to non-fallers with PD. This may be because of the difficulty in attention allocation and planning to coordinate successful movements necessary in walking.

There are also differences in how those with PD experience these cognitive deficits based on where their motor symptoms first developed. For instance, it has been reported that patients who developed motor symptoms on the right side of their body had greater working memory impairments compared to individuals who developed symptoms on their left side (Foster, Drago, Yung, Crucian, and Heilman, 2013). Reasons for this may have be the role of the left hemisphere in language functioning. Obeso and colleagues (2013) also observed a significant effect between cognitive dysfunction and side of development for motor symptom onset.

Interestingly the individual's level of impairment associated with their executive dysfunction can change as PD progresses. For instance, for planning tasks, patients with a mild degree of symptoms have been shown to not be as impaired on neuropsychological measures compared to those with more severe symptoms. As PD severity increased, individuals had significant increases in their processing speed, specifically with initiating correct responses and those with severe symptoms of PD demonstrated difficulty with response time, accuracy, and planning (Owen et al., 1992; Dirnberger and Jahanshai, 2013).

In considering the cognitive impairments associated with PD, it is not only important to recognize what they are but also to understand impact they may have on the individual's life. For instance, executive dysfunction has powerful implications for functional abilities and coping strategies (Kudlicka, Clare, and Hindle 2013). In this study, Kudlicka and colleagues (2013) administered measures such as quality of life satisfaction scale, the PD questionnaire, the caregiver burden questionnaire, and various neuropsychological assessments for evaluating executive functioning. Findings suggest a relationship between quality of life, health status, and executive functioning. Kudlicka and colleagues (2013) argued that executive dysfunction-related difficulties coupled with behavioral and emotional dysregulation directly impacted the quality of the patients' lives. This suggests that while patients with PD may receive some relief in various areas of executive functioning, it may worsen in others.

11.2 Huntington's Disease

Originally identified in 1872 by George Huntington as Huntington's chorea, Huntington's disease (HD) is a genetically inherited fatal neurodegenerative disorder with a triad of cognitive, motor, and psychiatric components (Group, 1993). Inheriting a dominant gene on Chromosome 4 of the IT-5 gene causes HD. This gene codes for the expression of the protein huntingtin, which has direct implications for motor coordination (Belinger et al., 2010). The prognosis after diagnosis is sixteen to seventeen years of life (Roos, Hermans, Vegler-van der Vlis, Van Ommen, and Brayn, 1993) and most deaths in HD are due to secondary causes such as cardiovascular disease, pneumonia, choking, and suicide (Conneally, 1984). HD is usually separated into five stages. The first stage encompasses newly diagnosed patients that do not yet have significant cognitive impairment or functional deficits in activities of daily living. Conversely, stage five of the disease is when symptoms are of such a severe nature that the patient cannot function independently and needs complete support in all activities of daily living (Conneally, 1984).

HD is estimated to occur in every 10 per 100,000 individuals, with the majority of the prevalence occurring in Whites (Novak and Tabrizi, 2005). There are no significant differences between genders for frequency of diagnosis (Conneally, 1984). The age of onset for first receiving an official diagnosis of HD can vary but is typically between 35 and 45 years (King et al., 2011; Novak and Tabrizi, 2010). Even though the majority of cases will fall within this range, there are still 10% of cases which qualify for late onset (diagnosis at age 50 or greater) or early-onset (diagnosis before age 20) (King et al., 2011).

11.2.1. Cognitive Impairments

Psychiatric symptoms and motor impairments comprise two aspects of the HD triumvirate for functional impairment. The last component of impairments is within the cognitive domain. Previous research suggests that cognitive impairment in those with HD includes psychomotor slowing, loss of memory, impaired free recall, difficulty concentrating, and executive dysfunction (Bonelli and Cummings, 2007; Montoya et al., 2006; King et al., 2011). Processing speed improved temporarily during the first year but soon dropped back to very low in the second year. Working memory and sustained attention saw improvements at the second testing time, but performance regressed back to the original classification of very low at the third testing time (King et al., 2011). Belinger and colleagues (2010) explored the progression of cognitive change using a variety of neuropsychological measures including the RBANS, Unified Huntington's Disease Rating Scale, and subtests of various measures. These included Digit Symbol Coding, Digit Span, figure copy, and memory tests including figure recall at two testing times across sixteen months. Their findings suggested a noticeable change in cognition in those with HD across a 16 month span, with psychomotor slowing and executive dysfunction present in the early stages of the disease with more diffuse and severe impairments occurring later. The main impairments with executive functioning include difficulties with set shifting, planning, and attention (Aron et al., 2003; Lawrence, Sahakian, Hodges, 1996; Lawrence, Sahakian, and Robbins, 1998; Belinger et al., 2010; King et al., 2011; Klempir et al., 2009; Allain et al., 2011, Eddy et al., 2012; Sprengelmeyer et al., 2013; Sitek et al., 2013).

11.2.2. Shifting deficits

Even when individuals are in the early stage of HD, they exhibit significantly poorer performance on measures evaluating shifting attention, specifically on tasks where an individual is asked to switch between two different tasks (Aron et al., 2003; Lawrence, Sahakian, and Hodges, 1996). Similar to how motor deficits in Parkinson's disease correlate with some of their cognitive impairments, HD research suggests that there may be a relationship between involuntary movements and executive dysfunction. Specifically, correlational analyses revealed that executive functioning manipulates voluntary movements, in other words, executive dysfunction serves as a mediator between involuntary movements and cognitive impairment (Klempir et al., 2009).

11.2.3. Updating deficits

Lawrence's research group (1996) found that people with HD exhibited poorer spatial working memory than that of controls. This means that these patients struggled with spatially updating information, such as abstractly being able to spatially picture a map and mentally reversing the route. Later stages of progression showed difficulties with simpler tasks such as reverse learning, but even at a very early stage of the disease a negative impact on spatial working memory was evident. This deficit could severely impact daily functioning, such as anticipating accurate spatial calculations required for pouring a cup of coffee or driving safely in traffic. The authors concluded that these deficiencies were related to the anatomical changes to the connectivity of the striatum that resulted from the neuropathological staging of the disease.

11.2.4. Inhibition deficits

Swerdlow and colleagues (2014) found that in addition to the interruption of the prepulse inhibition of both acoustic and tactile startle responses, the inhibitory control mechanism was hindered in a sample of people with HD. In addition to the inhibitory control deficit, the sensorimotor inhibition control, or gating, has been documented as deficient due to the striatal degeneration. This evidence was demonstrated when the HD patients did not exhibit prepulse inhibition after either acoustic or tactile stimuli. Even when the normal subjects exhibited maximum levels of gating, the patients with HD demonstrated little to no prepulse inhibition.

11.2.5. Impact

Another implication for the quality of their life rests on their lack of awareness into their cognitive difficulties. Sitek and colleagues (2013) gave several self-report questionnaires to individuals suffering from HD and matched them to caregiver questionnaires. Results revealed that self-awareness is impaired (Sitek et al., 2013). Mirroring this, Lagavant and colleagues (2012) found that individuals with HD also show impairment in awareness of memory difficulties and this effect was directly associated with disease severity, functional decline, motor dysfunction and executive dysfunction. More importantly this lack of insight, or anosognia, came about rather quickly in the progression of their disease as individuals with HD only stayed attuned to their difficulties during the early stages of the disease. Anosognosia may have powerful implications into caregiver burden and overall quality of life in individuals diagnosed with Huntington's disease.

In conclusion, Huntington's disease is a genetically inherited fatal neuro-degenerative disorder, which involves a variety of complex symptoms across the motor, psychiatric, and cognitive domains. The main symptoms include chorea and rigidity in motor impairments, depression and irritability in psychiatric impairments, and processing speed and executive dysfunction in cognitive impairments.

More specifically within executive dysfunction, patients exhibit difficulties with shifting attention, concentration, inhibition, planning, and theory of mind. Although they may have limited awareness of their deficits, these deficits all have important implications for the quality of their own lives while coping and managing the symptoms of their disease and the quality of their caregivers' lives. Currently, Huntington's disease is not curable, and its prognosis is terminal. How individuals and their caregivers cope with these deficits will enable those suffering with the disease to maximize quality of life.

11.3 Multiple Sclerosis

Multiple sclerosis (MS) is a chronic autoimmune disorder, most prominently marked by a loss of neural connections in the central nervous system. Within MS there are four possible subtypes. The first is relapsing-remitting (RRMS). This includes an acute worsening of symptoms followed by complete recovery and no progression of disability. The second possible subtype of the disease is secondary progressive (SPMS) or a progressive worsening of neurological functioning with only minor improvements. The third possible subtype is labeled primary progressive (PPMS) and is when there is a progression of symptoms continuously from the disease onset. The last subtype is progressive-relapsing (PRMS), which involves a steady worsening of symptoms from onset and a variable degree of recovery. The first two subtypes RRMS and SPMS are the most common with SPMS resulting the greatest cognitive impairment (DeLuca, Chelune, Tulsky, Lengenfelder, and Chiaravalloti, 2004; DeLuca and Nocentini, 2011).

The two main neurobiological processes involved are demyelination and axonal damage (DeLuca and Nocentini, 2011). Neurons in the brain are coated with myelin sheaths that essentially serve as insulators around the axon to allow for faster conduction. When this casing degrades or becomes damaged, the neuronal signal cannot get passed down the axon as quickly or efficiently. Thus the myelin sheath is an integral part of information processing and executive deficits in MS. Additional research suggests that MS involves plaques and lesions in the brain and spinal cord. The plaques are widespread throughout the brain and their diffuse distribution may account for the variety of impairments in those with MS (Chiaravalloti and DeLuca, 2008).

The disease is estimated to occur in 400,000 people in the United States and 2.1 million people worldwide (Deluca and Nocentini, 2011). Research has found correlations between geographic location and prevalence of those suffering from MS. Specifically, in northern Europe there exists a frequency of 100 individuals per 100,000 compared to other regions with lower rates, such as Asia and Africa (Kurtzke, 2000). Mirroring this geographic pattern, MS is most common in those of northern European ancestry though it can occur in all races (Motl, Arnett, Smith, Barack, Benedict, and Ahlstrom, 2008; Chiaravalloti, and DeLuca, 2008). MS is more common in females than in males (DeLuca and Nocentini, 2011). Age of onset is typically between 20 and 40 years (DeLuca and Nocentini, 2011; Reingold, 1995). While the majority of patients fall within this range, 10% experience early onset with 2.1% of individuals with MS diagnosed before the age of sixteen years old (Ekmecki, Yuckeyar, and Sagduyu, 2012). Late onset of symptoms can also occur after the age of fifty years (DeLuca, Chelune, Tulsky, Longenfelder, and Chiaravalloti, 2011).

11.3.1. Cognitive impairment

In addition to motor and psychiatric symptoms, those with MS experience cognitive impairments, with rates as high as 65% reported for cognitive difficulties in MS (Staples and Lincoln, 1979). The cognitive impairments in MS include dysfunction in the following areas: complex attention, information processing speed, verbal memory, visual memory, learning/forgetfulness, distractibility, attention span, and executive functioning (Amato et al, 2014). Specific executive functioning deficits include difficulty in completing tasks, initiating new tasks when other tasks are incomplete, abstract reasoning, verbal fluency, organization, planning, and problem solving (Pierson and Griffith, 2006; Amato et al., 2014; Brassington and Marsh, 1998; Bagert, Caplair, Bourdette, 2002; Bobholz and Rao, 2003). Pierson and Giffith (2006) suggested that the main cause of executive dysfunction in MS is buildup of plaques and demylination of the neurons in the frontal lobe.

Cognitive impairment can be observed early in MS and then progresses over the course of the disease depending on the subtype (Faiss, 2007). In order to elucidate changes in cognitive impairment overtime, Achiron and colleagues (2013) looked at the trajectory of cognitive impairment across 30 years. They found that the biggest cognitive impairments were in processing speed and executive functions. At the 5-year mark, 20% of MS patients out of a sample of 1500 performed 1 standard deviation (SD) below the mean on the cognitive tasks and 6% performed below 2 SD. At 10 years, this worsened to 29.3% of individuals with MS performing 1 SD below and 9% 2 SD below the mean (Archiron, et al., 2013).

Basso and colleagues (2008) used the Frontal Systems Behavioral Scale (FrSBe) to measure self-reported dysexecutive symptoms in MS. They also found significant differences on objective performance-based measures such as TMT parts A and B and the California Verbal Learning Test-II between MS patients and healthy controls. Self-report symptoms of executive dysfunction correlated with actual executive dysfunction. This suggests that these individuals had relatively good awareness into their difficulties.

In contrast, Goverover, Chairavalloti, and DeLuca (2005) found that self-awareness of symptoms is inversely related to the extent of their cognitive impairment. They reported that measures of executive dysfunction, disinhibition, and apathy were negatively correlated with self-awareness of executive dysfunction. Mirroring this, other studies regarding insight to awareness of deficits of MS report that individuals were less aware of their cognitive deficits when executive dysfunction was high (Smith and Arnett, 2010)

11.3.2. Shifting deficits

Attentional deficits have been noted in patients with MS by Dujardin, Donze, and Hautecouer (2003). Early in the progression of the disease, cognitive loading yielded findings that patients demonstrated a deficit in processing resources. Without compensating their existing attentional mechanisms, these patients performed at a significantly lower level of attending when compared to their healthy peers. Another study by MacAllister and colleagues (2005) demonstrated that shifting attention between stimuli was particularly hindered in nearly one-third of patients diagnosed with MS. Chiaravalloti and DeLuca (2008) further emphasized the daily tasks impeded by deficits in complex attention, which include maintaining employment.

11.3.3. Updating deficits

Chiaravalloti and DeLuca (2005) also discussed the working memory deficits that further complicate daily tasks for patients with MS, such as managing a household. Amato and colleagues (1995) reported additional findings of working memory deficits, including abstract reasoning, which negatively impacted their prognosis and independence in daily living. Ultimately, a life already complicated by constant pain and medical ailments is further detrimented by incrementally increasing deficits in simultaneous mental capacities.

11.3.4. Inhibition deficits

To further complicate an already distressful situation, Deloire and colleagues (2004) also noted statistically significant impairments in inhibition in a sample of people with MS. It is important to note that the level of impairment was reflective of the tissue damage due to lesions associated with the disease. This means that the more severe the physical damage due to the deleterious effects of the disease, the more intensive inhibitory setbacks a person with MS would experience.

11.3.5. Impact

As noted throughout this section, individuals with MS experience a variety of cognitive deficits. Unfortunately, these deficits have substantial implications for quality of life and caregiver burden. Cognitive dysfunction can impact physical independence, employment, social and recreational activities, driving skills, physical rehabilitation, and caregiver strain. For example, 40-80% of people with MS are unemployed (Gronning, Hannisdal, and Mellgren, 1990; Kornblith, LaRoca, and Baum, 1996). Krause and colleagues (2013) conducted a study comparing motor, psychiatric, and cognitive symptoms among unemployed and employed people with MS. Their findings indicated that those in the unemployed group illustrated greater elevations in neurological disability, depressive symptoms, fatigue, and significantly lower cognitive functioning.

11.4. HIV

Human immunodeficiency virus (HIV) is a chronic disease that spreads through bodily fluids and attacks specific cells, such as CD4 cells and T-cells, in the immune system (Center of Disease Control and Prevention, 2013). HIV is treatable but uncurable and can lead to acquired immunodeficiency syndrome (AIDS). AIDS is the advanced and more severe level of HIV. The HIV virus can lead to many complications, including infection of the central nervous system (CNS) leading to neurological problems (Vance, Fazeli, Moneyham, Keltner, and Raper, 2013). When HIV causes neurological deficits, it is referred to as HIV-associated neurological disorders (HAND).

Though other neurological problems exist regardless of a HAND diagnosis, there are three common subtypes of HAND in patients diagnosed with the virus: Asymptomatic Neurocognitive Impairment (ANI), Mild Neurocognitive Disorder (MND), and HIV-Associated Dementia (HAD; Center of Disease Control and Prevention, 2013). ANI is the most common and least impairing. It causes mild neurocognitive impairment without significant functional impairment. MND is more impairing, causing mild to moderate difficulties in at least two cognitive domains and mild impairment in daily functioning. HAD, otherwise known as HIV-encephalopathy or HIV

Dementia complex, is the most severe of these HAND subtypes (Encephalitis Society, 2013). HAD causes moderate to severe impairments in at least two areas of cognition with significant impairments in daily living that are not fully explainable by other comorbidities such as delirium. HAD is also associated with impairments in movement, such as bradykinesia, as well as bradyphrenia (slowed information processing) (Woods, Moore, Weber, and Grant, 2009).

About 50,000 people are infected with HIV each year in the United States. It is estimated that 1.1 million people are infected with HIV in the United States (CDC, 2012). Of this number, 18% are not aware of their status. A nationwide survey was initiated in 1988 to measure HIV prevalence in childbirths (Gwinn et al., 1991). This 1989 survey included 38 states and one province, which resulted in an estimated 1.5 per 1000 women giving birth to infants infected with HIV. Their estimates yielded an approximation of 1800 newborns infected with HIV during that 12-month period.

11.4.1. Cognitive impairments

Children diagnosed with perinatal HIV have been shown to differ from age-related uninfected peers in several areas of cognition. It has been reported that they perform worse on processing speed and visuospatial tasks and have impairments in executive functioning (Laughton, Cornell, Boivin, and Van Rie, 2013). The most consistent finding in children and adolescents with HIV has been problems with attention and expressive language, which can be considered executive in nature. These deficits are pervasive and can cause symptoms similar to Autism Spectrum Disorder (Landry and Smith, 1998; Mitchell, 2001; Woods, Moore, Weber, and Grant, and 2009). As the disease progresses, adolescents can display symptoms similar to HAD (Mitchell, 2001). However, these deficits are dependent on the severity of HIV progression (Landry and Smith, 1998; Mitchell, 2001; Laughton, Cornell, Boivin, and Van Rie, 2013). In particular, the presence of encephalopathy has significant implications for their cognitive deficits. Children and adolescence diagnosed with HIV without encephalopathy typically perform very similarly to their uninfected peers. Understanding the levels of encephalopathy associated with HIV is important in understanding the level of neurocognitive impairment in children.

Encephalopathy is common in HIV. There are two types: progressive and static. Progressive is the most prevalent form and is further divided into three categories: subacute, plateau, and static. Subacute progressive encephalopathy is associated with developmental regression in children and severe deficits in cognition, motor, social-emotional, adaptive functioning, and linguistics.

Plateau progressive encephalopathy is less severe and refers to limited developmental gains. Static encephalopathy allows a patient to continue to gain skill but at a lower rate than would be expected for that individual's age (Landry and Smith, 1998). Understanding a child's level of impairment, including their type of encephalopathy, can allow teachers to better adjust teaching the child at the appropriate level and reduce the poorer school performance often observed in students with HIV (Laughton, Cornell, Boivin, and Van Rie, 2013).

It is important to note that highly active antiretroviral therapy can reverse HIV-related neurocognitive impairment, the neuropsychological deficits may persist (Valerio et al., 2007). The most common comorbidities associated with HIV have been documented as oral candidiasis (21%), peripheral neuropathy (16%), and the mean number of HIV and medical comorbidities was 1.1, which did not differ by age. In this particular study by Kilbourne, Justice, Rabeneck, Rodriguez-Barradas, and Weissman (2001), the mean age was 49 years and 54% of their sample identified as African-American. Furthermore, 46% exhibited depressive symptoms, 32% anxiety, and 11% cognitive impairment.

11.4.2. Shifting deficits

Cognitive impairments have been repeatedly noted in patients with HIV, particularly in HIV-seropositive individuals (Farinpour et al., 2000; Koekkoek, de Sonneville, Wolfs, Licht, and Geelen, 2007; Martin et al., 2001). Specifically, shifting attention, which allows a person to switch focus between multiple stimuli such as a ringing phone and answering the door, was one of the most impaired executive functions in children with HIV compared to healthy controls (Koekkoek, de Sonneville, Wolfs, Licht, and Geelen, 2007).

11.4.3. Updating deficits

Koekkoek and colleagues (2007) also cited working memory as one of the most impaired cognitive function in patients with HIV, particularly visuospatial working memory. Stout et al. (1995) additionally described working memory declines as positively incrementally associated with the progression of HIV infection. Namely, they found processing speed did not significantly differ as previous researchers had (Koekkoek, de Sonneville, Wolfs, Licht, and Geelen, 2007), but that working memory declines were still evident despite no changes in processing speed. This would indicate that these deficits are largely due to aspects of working memory outside of processing speed, which was previously touted as a main contributor to the changes. The updating deficits were significant, particularly for symptomatic HIV+ individuals. They also concluded that the noticeable decline probably begins during the asymptomatic phase, which means early detection and arrangements for future preparations are an important change that must occur early in the progression of the infection.

Furthermore, Farinpour and colleagues (2000) found similar results: Working memory deficits were more frequent in symptomatic participants, particularly within HIV-seropositive people. However, this study examined verbal working memory as visuospatial working memory had been documented previously. As such, their conclusion was that working memory deficits were in fact not domain-specific. Again, HIV+ subjects were measured to perform significantly worse than their controls in the working memory domain (Martin et al., 2001). This particular evaluation of working memory was different in that it involved auditory working memory.

11.4.4. Inhibition deficits

Inhibition deficits have been noted in patients with HIV, and have been noted as both cognitive (Moran, Booze, and Mactutus, 2006) and sensorimotor (Minassian et al., 2013) in nature. Moran, Booze, and Mactutus (2006) found that almost half of HIV-1-positive subjects on therapy were afflicted with HAND. In exploring these impairments in rats, the primary deficits noted were executive functions, including inhibition. Minassian and colleagues (2013) found that the ability to filter out irrelevant information was hindered in individuals with HIV. More significantly, individuals with HAND exhibited more severe deficits in prepulse inhibition.

11.4.5. Comorbidities

As a patient with HIV ages, more neurological problems arise. Not only are the neurological issues associated with HIV prevalent, but also CNS-opportunistic infections increase (Price et al., 1988; Grant and Heaton, 1990; Simpson and Tagliati, 1994). Similarly to children and adolescents, adults with HIV also demonstrate deficits in executive functions, like processing speed, attention, language and psychomotor ability, learning, abstraction, memory, and working memory (Grant and Heaton, 1990; Chang et al., 2004; Woods, Moore, Weber, and Grant, 2009; Vance, Fazeli, Moneyham, Keltner, and Raper, 2013). HIV dementia is more common in adults with HIV than children, which causes problems with forgetfulness, cognition, psychomotor slowing, impaired concentration, and coordination (Grant and Heaton, 1990; Vance, Fazeli, Moneyham, Keltner, and Raper, 2013). There is evidence of impaired neuronal plasticity, which is the ability of the CNS to respond to injury and promote the recovery of functioning. Loss of neurons and their branches are more common as the disease progresses (Avdoshina, Bachis, and Mocchetti, 2013).

Opportunistic infections of the CNS are common in adults with HIV. Such infections include CNS lymphoma, toxoplasma encephalitis, and vacuolar myelopathy (Price et al., 1988; Simpson and Tagliati, 1994). These infections contribute to impairment in cognitive domains as well as compounding the symptoms with headaches, memory loss, confusion, seizures, and urinary dysfunction (Simpson and Tagliati, 1994).

11.5 Spina Bifida

Spina bifida (SB) is a neural tube defect where the neural tube does not close and the backbone that protects the spinal cord does not fully form. Spina bifida affects about 1,500 births each year in the United States and is actually cited as the leading birth defect that causes permanent disability (Spina Bifida Association of America, 2014). According to Williams, Rasmussen, Flores, Kirby, and Edmonds (2005), SB rates are highest in Hispanic, then non-Hispanic white, before non-Hispanic black people. The overall prevalence rate of SB decreased significantly (31%; Williams et al., 2002) due to mandated folic acid consumption beginning in 1998. Due to recent advances in treatment, three-quarters of individuals with SB survive into adulthood with the exact life expectancy still unclear. There are several types of spina bifida, but the three most common types include spina bifida occulta, meningocele, and myelomeningocele (Center for Disease Control, 2013). Spina bifida occulta is the least impairing, also known as "hidden" SB; there is a small gap in the spine, but the spinal cord and nerves are normal and there are no risks of disabilities. Meningocele is caused when a fluid sac forms outside the spine, but the spinal cord and nerves are not exposed. That is when there is little to no evident damage. When referring to spina bifida, most people refer to myeloningocele, the most severe form. Myelomeningocele is when a fluid-like sac containing the spinal cord and nerves forms outside of the spine. This type of SB causes the most damage and a variety of disabilities.

Myelomeningocele (MMC), depending on its location on the spine, can cause partial to full paralysis (Center for Disease Control, 2013). People affected by MMC often have difficulties walking. Some people have little to no assistance in walking, and others have to use crutches, walkers, or wheelchairs. The level of mobility assistance required is dependent on the location of the sac. The higher up on the spine, the more disabled a person's mobility. Most people with MMC cannot control when they go to the bathroom, and often develop urinary tract infections. The vast majority of MMC cases are accompanied by hydrocephalus or water in or surrounding the brain. Hydrocephalus is treated by shunting to relieve pressure on the brain (Center for Disease Control, 2013). Half of MMC cases are also diagnosed with Chiari malformation type 2, a deformity of the cerebellum and brainstem. These brain deformities adversely affect development, resulting in neurological and cognitive deficits (Stubberud and Riemer, 2012).

11.5.1. Cognitive impairment

In several studies comparing performance in children with and without MMC, children with the disorder obtained low average full scale IQs (Soare and Raimondi, 1977; Zachary, 1977; Wills, Holmbeck, Dillon, and McLone, 1988; Casari and Fantino, 1998) but performed significantly lower on Performance IQ subtests than matched controls and had deficits in arithmetic and visuomotor functioning tests (Stubberud and Riemer, 2012). Those with shunted hydrocephalus performed lower on Performance IQ than unshunted and non-hyrdrocephalic individuals (Soare and Raimondi, 1977; Casari and Fantino, 1998) suggesting that the presence of hydrocephalus results in more significant cognitive impairments.

Nonverbal abilities undergo more deficits than verbal abilities in MMC individuals. As people with MMC increase in age, their rate of accruing new skills slows in comparison to their peers, especially on tests of arithmetic and visuomotor skills. Even so, performance on tests of reading and spelling skills seems to reflect typical development (Wills, Holmbeck, Dillon, and McLone, 1988). MMC performance deficits could be due to deficiencies in motor skills caused by associated physical disabilities.

Executive dysfunction has been shown to mediate the relationship between child dependency, intrinsic motivation, and adaptation skills (Kelly et al., 2012; Tuminello, Holmbeck, and Olson, 2012). Executive deficits result in problems with planning, accounting for consequences of actions, and making real-time adjustments, which can account deficits in psychosocial adaptation seen in SB (Stubberud and Reimer, 2012). These complications begin in childhood and adolescence and can continue to progress into adulthood affecting social relationships as well employment. Even for individuals with SB who have normal intelligence, learning difficulties have been noted (Spina

Bifida Association of America, 2014) which may reflect executive dysfunction.

11.5.2. Shifting deficits

Several studies have provided evidence for attentional and executive dysfunctions associated with MMC. Individuals diagnosed with MMC in childhood have exhibited deficits in attention as well as certain aspects of executive functioning. Children with MMC have showed deficiencies in attention, inhibition, and problem solving (Fletcher et al., 1996; Burmeister et al., 2005). These executive dysfunctions have been shown to continue into adulthood. More specifically, in comparison to ADHD, individuals with MMC displayed deficits in specific attention orienting tasks, such as inhibition of return and difficulty disengaging attention while those with ADHD typically exhibit deficits in sustained attention. People with MMC have normal performance on tasks of sustained attention and do not respond to stimulant medication, a commonly prescribed treatment for ADHD (Dennis and Barnes, 2010).

11.5.3. Updating deficits

When compared to healthy controls, working memory was impaired in patients both with or without hydrocephalus (Mammarella, Cornoldi, and Donadello, 2003). Again, the degree of impairment is important to note. These researchers found that working memory was increasingly impaired in increments related to hydrocephalus. More specifically, visual working memory deficits were noted in children with SB in a study that compared the performance on a specific visual discriminability that requires specific stimuli processing (Iddon, Morgan, Loveday, Sahakian, and Pickard, 2004).

11.5.4. Inhibition deficits

Children with MMC have poorer metacognitive skills than unaffected children (Kelly et al., 2012). They generally demonstrate poor planning abilities and difficulty shifting attention, focusing, and inhibiting impulses (Wills, 1993). Adolescents with this disorder also display significant deficits compared to controls in the areas of inhibition, initiation, sustained attention, and working memory as well as slower performance on executive functioning tasks, such as planning, sequencing, switching attention, and mental flexibility (Fletcher et al., 1996; Burmeister et al., 2005; Rose and Holmbeck, 2007; Tuminello, Holmbeck, and Olson, 2012). Similarly, adults with MMC also exhibit low inhibition, poor impulse control, impaired mental flexibility, and reduced working memory (Stubberud and Riemer, 2012). It should be noted that research in adults with MMC is limited.

As previously mentioned, people diagnosed with MMC often additionally suffer from hydrocephalus. Most of the studies examining deficits in attention and executive functioning have also analyzed the differences in these areas in spina bifida with and without hydrocephalus. Studies indicated that spina bifida with hydrocephalus (SBH) causes more deficits in executive functioning when compared to patients without SBH and normal controls (Wills, 1993; Iddon, Morgan, Loveday, Sahakian, and Pickard, 2004 Burmeister et al. 2005; Rose and Holmbeck, 2007; Tuminello, Holmbeck, and Olson, 2012). People with SBH who received a shunt procedure performed significantly worse on measures of executive functioning (Wills, 1993; Fletcher et al., 1996; Iddon, Morgan, Loveday, Sahakian, and Pickard, 2004; Burmeister et al., 2005; Rose and Holmbeck, 2007; Kelly et al., 2012; Tuminello, Holbeck, and Olson, 2012). It is likely that executive dysfunction is exacerbated by the shunting procedure, seizures, infections, and the additional reconstruction of the shunts required throughout the lifespan (Snow et al., 1994; Brown et al., 2008).

11.5.5. Impact

Deficits in executive function in patients with SB affect them not only academically, but socially as well. Several studies have shown correlations between executive dysfunctions associated with SB and maladaptive psychosocial skills (Kelly et al., 2012; Stubberud and Reimer, 2012; Tuminello, Holmbeck, and Olson, 2012). Children and adolescents with SB who experience more executive dysfunction tend to be less independent and socially adapt than those with higher executive functioning and normal peers (Rose and Holmbeck, 2007; Heffelfinger et al., 2008; Tuminello, Holmbeck, and Olson, 2012). The Spina Bifida Association of America (2014) reported that most adults with SB have difficulties living independently due to a number of factors including poor problem-solving likely related to updating and shifting deficits that inhibit using new approaches to problems, self/family beliefs and perceptions, and social isolation.

11.6. Alzheimer's Disease

The progression of Alzheimer's disease (AD) is gradual, and has been recorded to last anywhere from two years to twenty (BrightFocus Foundation, 2014). This progressive deterioration of mental capacities has been linked with many biological and external risk and protective factors. Clark and colleagues (2013) compared the subtypes of mild cognitive impairment to the conventional diagnostic models and found that some of these prodromal subtypes could possibly serve as false-positives, though this has yet to be replicated. The physical biomarkers related to AD exist well in advance of the symptoms. This progression of the disease has been labeled with stages, which include a pre-clinical, prodromal, and dementia stages including mild, moderate, and severe stages. The prodromal stage has been identified as an intermediate condition of memory loss with the severity of loss ranked between normal aging and dementia. The actual stages of dementia due to AD include mild AD, which is usually characterized by impaired learning of new information and possible mood swings. The second stage, moderate AD, is characterized by more severe impairments in memory, executive functioning, and visuospatial abilities and a noticeable impairment in functional independence. Severe AD, the last category, involves severe cognitive impairments, behavioral comorbidities, and physical deterioration resulting in the need for constant care. Diagnosis. In order to be diagnosed with AD, a patient must undergo several components of an interdisciplinary exam. Most people present with initial memory complaints. A physician will perform a physical examination to rule out other physical etiologies and refers to a neuropsychologist for testing to objectively measure cognitive symptoms and rule out other contributions. The diagnostic criteria include evidence of cognitive decline from a previous level, particularly in attention, executive functioning, learning and memory, language, perceptual-motor, or social cognition as described by a respondent or cognitive performance (APA, 2013). These deficits must interfere with everyday activities, are not due to delirium or other mental disorders, and there is a gradual progression of at least one cognitive domain. Additionally, either genetic evidence of AD or a clear decline in memory and learning, a gradual decline in cognition, and an absence of other neurological explanations is required.

According to Beeri, Werner, Davidson, and Noy (2000), the behavioral and psychological symptoms of dementia totaled an additional annual indirect cost of $2,665 and additional annual direct cost was of $1,450 more than the total annual direct cost. The behaviors and psychiatric symptoms they included were hallucinations, delusions, depression, euphoria, agitation, aggression, abnormal vocalizations, wandering, over-activity, sexual disinhibition, sleep disturbances, and apathy. Mega, Cummings, Fiorello, and Gornbein (1996) reported similar behaviors, including delusions, hallucinations, agitation, dysphoria, anxiety, euphoria, apathy, disinhibition, irritability, and aberrant motor behavior. Burns, Jacoby, and Levy (1990) studied the percentages of patients with reported potentially hazardous and emotionally straining clinical behaviors in patients with AD: urinary incontinence (48%), aggression (20), wandering (19%), binge-eating (10%), hyperorality (6%), and sexual disinhibition (7%). The psychiatric deficits associated with AD may offer a potentially viable mode for increasing independence in AD. Specifically, psychiatric impairments were correlated more positively and significantly with institutionalization when compared to cognitive deficits as predictors.

Nearly half of all dementia cases are accounted for by AD (Weintraub, Wicklund, and Salmon, 2012). According to Hebert and colleagues (2013), AD prevalence rates were estimated 11% over the age of 65 years. The rate increases with age and over 85 years of age, about half of individuals have probable AD. The American Psychiatric Association (2013) echoed this steep prevalence increase by age. The general prevalence rate of the population for people over 65 years was reported to range from 2% to 30%.

11.6.1. Cognitive Impairments

Cognitive impairments have been documented as heterogeneous manifestations in groups with AD and mild cognitive impairment (Tatsuoka et al., 2013), though the classic presentation is predominantly amnestic in nature. Specific cognitive profiles have been associated with the differential rates of AD. This indicates the noticeable cognitive change evident even before conversion to AD from mild impairment. AD cognitive deficits are not limited to executive functions, but also include more broad descriptions of attention, processing speeds, and most notably, deficits in memory.

11.6.2. Shifting deficits

Individuals with AD are reportedly impaired on measures of divided, selective, and sustained attention (Perry and Hodges, 1998). Modeled after lesion studies and functional imaging, attentional control was particularly impaired in domains that involved set-shifting. This deficit was apparent even in the earlier stages of AD when sustained attention was preserved. Calderon and colleagues (2000) compared performances on executive tasks by patients with dementia with Lewy bodies (DLB) and with AD. Though the DLB patients were significantly more impaired on global attention measures, AD patients showed deficits in selective attention and set shifting in particular.

11.6.3. Updating deficits

Working memory deficits have been noted throughout the Alzheimer's literature (Baddeley, Bressi, Sala, Logie, and Spinnler, 1991; Collette, Van der Linden, Bechet, Belleville, and Salmon, 1997). These deficits in working memory have been explored in relation to memory when compared to both healthy controls (Baddeley et al., 1986), and when compared to previous performance with the self as the control comparison (Baddeley, Bressi, Sala, Logie, and Spinnler, 1991). Collette, Van der Linden, Bechet, Belleville, and Salmon (1997) found that working memory was significantly impaired compared to elderly controls when the task involved recall and alphabetization of a series of words. Interestingly, these researchers also concluded that not all components of working memory were affected, as demonstrated by similar performance across groups on a dual task involving digits and a visuomotor task. That said, it was noted that many of the components involved in updating functions were impaired to a degree that it would negatively impact daily functioning.

11.6.4. Inhibition deficits

Belanger, Belleville, and Gauthier (2009) evaluated inhibition in patients with AD and compared it to inhibitory performances by people with mild cognitive impairment (MCI), healthy older adults, and younger adults. These researchers used sections of the Stroop effect with results that indicated reduced resistance to interfering stimuli, even significantly worse than the impairments noted in MCI and healthy older adults.

11.6.5. Impact

The symptoms previously described depict a life of independence grossly interrupted by cognitive dysfunction, which can mar social interactions, daily living, and even has been correlated with physical impairments. Additionally, the psychiatric symptoms that are often comorbid with AD result in higher rates of institutionalization. These findings hint at a more individualized approach to understanding the course of AD: people experience different rates of decline, different types of decline, and therefore have a vastly heterogeneous history.

In consideration of the cognitive impairments associated with AD, it is imperative to acknowledge not only the scientific definitions of these deficits, but to truly consider the impact these deficiencies have on a person cognitively, emotionally, and functionally. Additionally, there are often significant negative physical changes, as well as economic and overall declines. This is a disease that has an everlasting impact on the caretakers and individuals and progressively seeps into every domain of daily living.

12. Broad Impact of Executive Dysfunction

As we discussed, executive impairments associated with neurological disorders are not only constructs defined for research, but also real factors that negatively impact patients' quality of life and self-care. These people have multifaceted lives that are complicated by varying degrees of medical, motor, psychiatric, and cognitive issues that interfere with their independence. This section reviews the impact of executive dysfunction from an individualized perspective.

12.1. Impact on the individual

Executive abilities refer to fluid cognitive skills that help use to adjust to and accommodate everyday tasks. The individual with Parkinson's Disease (PD), many experience tremors and may be dependent on some motor assistance. In addition to experiencing depression, hopelessness, and a sense of betrayal that their body will not cooperate, this patient may have to rely completely on others to pay their bills or to verify the correct amount of change at the grocery store. These issues are real world updating impairments. Updating could also refer to something as simple as remembering if a person has already showered for the day, or which body part has already been washed.

Executive dysfunction includes deficits in planning. Proper organization results from healthy executive functioning. For populations that have chronic medical conditions like HIV, planning plays an important role in attending required medical appointments and medication management. Additionally, organizing transportation is a common necessity for individuals with physical and motor ailments. If a person struggled with shifting attention, they could have significant difficulty driving as driving is a complex task that requires constantly shift between external cues (Gronning, Hannisdal, and Mellgren, 1990).

Kudlicka, Clare, and Hindle (2013) posited that executive dysfunction, particularly deficits in inhibition, exhibited a direct impact on patients' quality of life ratings. Inhibitory issues are relatively common in neurological disorders. In patients with Huntington's, these effects of disinhibition are evident early in the development of the disease (Lawrence, Sahakian, Hodges, 1996). Neurologic populations show higher rates of gambling, riskier sexual encounters, medically relevant weight gain, smoking, and/or rates of drug use. As an example, spina bifida is known to have a direct link with increased levels of obesity (Spina Bifida Association of America, 2014). King and colleagues (2011) reported that executive dysfunction is often chronic in these populations and any improvements are often short-term.

12.2. Socially

Each of these factors (or combination of factors) not only shapes this individual's life, it impacts how that person interacts with others. For example, a parent who experiences significant updating deficits may easily forget tasks such as picking up children from school (Gioia and Isquith, 2004). Other difficulties associated with updating involve concentration deficits and staying on task. Remaining on task is important in social situations. Individuals diagnosed with neurological disorders rely on social support. However, relationships are reciprocal and require that patients engage with their friends. One example of this would involve active listening, which would be detrimentally affected if updating were impaired.

Suhr (1997) reported that impaired inhibitory control was a predictive marker for entering a psychotic state and poorer coping skills. Additionally, deficits in shifting attention have been indicated in rigidity (Gioia and Isquith, 2004). Often, this is expressed as extreme difficulties with learning new approaches at work and in school and may result emotional outbursts related to new situations or changes in plans. This would hinder not only daily emotional stability for the individual, but also those close to this person, those who may have to interact with the person, like medical professionals or even employers.

Many studies have reported social deficits in populations diagnosed with neurological disorders, particularly in people who experience noticeable executive dysfunction (Gorerover, et al., 2005; Gronning, Hannisdal, and Mellgren, 1990; Krause, et al., 2013). One common negative behavior associated with a deficit in inhibition is constant interruption of others. For a person with executive dysfunction, this easily could complicate social interactions. If social support is hindered then emotional, financial, and functional stability could also suffer related to dissolution of relationships.

12.3. Burden

Individuals diagnosed with neurological disorders often have increased rates of executive dysfunction, psychiatric symptoms, and frequency of medical appointments. These issues may negatively influence family dynamics. An affected parent may be less likely to plan out being able to attend family events, such as school plays or soccer games. Unemployment is also a frequent complication and can further strain the family. These issues may result in the patient feeling like a burden on their children, spouse, or parents. Joiner (2009) described this as perceived burdensomeness. His theory of suicidal behavior posits that coupled with the sensation of being excluded (thwarted belongingness, potentially due to decreased attendance of family events), suicidal ideation would increase in this type of patient.

From a systems level approach, this patient could experience guilt in addition to familial obligations. Potentially, they may feel a compounded shame concerning diagnosis, required assistance, increased medical attention, and possibly as if they contribute less to the community overall. Executive dysfunction also has a financial impact, though there is little research quantifying the exact amount. For example, obesity, drug use, MS, diabetes, and dementia all have reported financial and ecological costs that are reported each year (Center for Disease Control, 2014). However, it is unknown what the contribution of executive dysfunction specifically is to these numbers.

Gioia and Isquith (2004) have criticized current assessment methods of executive functions as being insensitive and ecologically invalid. Instead, they emphasized the necessity of understanding family stress, resources, and caregiver coping skills in order to provide appropriate interventions related to executive issues. In addition to the neuropsychological measures currently used to define specific deficits, these researchers advocated for assessment that would involve the quantification of the behavioral manifestations outside the evaluation that result from these dysfunctions as well as the system-level factors that interact with the executive dysfunction. This area of research is significantly lacking. It is imperative to understand how these difficulties influence people's adaptive functions. In order to arrive at this improved method of evaluation, first healthcare providers will need to report the systemic level, financial, and daily cost of executive dysfunction.

CONCLUSION

The negative effects of executive dysfunction we described throughout this review focused on impaired shifting, updating, and inhibition components of the more global executive construct. Though these include only three underlying executive functions, they affect many aspects of a person's daily functioning including emotional, cognitive, and social aspects. We have demonstrated that core components of executive abilities have wide ranging effects on daily functioning. Additionally, this area of research is relatively scant compared to its tremendous real world impact and further study is needed. It is our experience than physicians frequently overestimate executive functioning in neurologic patients or at least assume sufficiently intact executive abilities for tasks such as medication management and medical decision making, often without any formal evaluation. This is problematic when specific patient populations are known to have executive impairments that will interfere with planning, judgment, and decision making as well as generally negatively affect quality of life. Hopefully, this review will act to inform healthcare professionals, caregivers, and family members of these relatively common issues in patients with neurologic conditions and lead to understanding and appropriate intervention.

REFERENCES

Aarnoudse-Moens, C. S. H., Weisglas-Kuperus, N., Duivenvoorden, H. J., Oosterlaan, J., and van Goudoever, J. B. (2012). Neonatal and parental predictors of executive function in very preterm children. *Acta Paediatrica*, 102, 282 – 286. doi: 10.1111/apa.12101

Aarsland, D., Bronnick, K., Alves, G., Tsynes, O., Pederson, K., Ehrt, U., and Larsen, J.P. (2009). The spectrum of neuropsychiatric symptoms inpatients with early untreated Parkinson's disease. *Journal of Neurology, Neurosurgery* and Psychiatry, 80, 928-930.

Aarsland, D., and Kurz., M. (2010). The Epidemiology associated with Parkinson's Disease. *Brain Pathology*, 20, 633-639. doi: 10.1111/j.1750-3639.2009.00369.

Achiron, A., Chapman, J., Magalashvilli, D., Dolev, M., Lavie, M., Bercovich, E., Polliack, M., Doniger, G.M., Stern, Y., Khilkevich, O., Menascu, S., Hararai, G., Gurevich, M., and Barak, Y. (2013). Modeling of cognitive impairment by disease duration in multiple sclerosis: A cross-sectional study. *PLoS One*, 8,1-11.

Adrover-Roig, D., Sese, A., Barcelo, F., and Palmer, A. (2012). A latent variable approach to executive control in healthy ageing. *Brain and Cognition*, 78, 284-289. doi:10.1016/j.bandc.2012.01.005

Allain, P., Havet-Thomassin, V., Verny, C., Gohier, B., and Lancelot, C. (2011). Evidence for deficits on different components of theory of mind in Huntington's disease. *Neuropsychiatry,* 25, 741-751. DOI: 10.1037/a0024408.

Allcock, L. M., Rowan, E. N., Steen, I. N., Wesnes, K., Kenny, R. A., and Burn, D. J. (2009). Impaired attention predicts falling in Parkinson's disease. *Parkinsonism and Related Disorders*, 15(2), 110-115.

Amato, M., Goretti, B., Viterbo, R., Portaccio, E., Niccolai, C., Hakiki, B., Iaffaldano, P., and Trojano, M. (2014). Computer assisted rehabilitation of attention in patients with Multiple Sclerosis: results of a randomized double blind trial. *Multiple Sclerosis Journal*, 20, 91-98. DOI: 10.1177 /1352458513501571

Amato, M., Ponziani, G., Pracucci, G., Bracco, L., Siracusa, G., and Amaducci, L. (1995). Cognitive impairment in early-onset multiple sclerosis: Pattern, predictors, and impact on everyday life in a 4-year follow-up. *Archives of Neurology,* 52(2), 168-172. doi:10.1001/archneur.1995.00540260072019

American Psychiatric Association. (2013). Diagnostic and Statistical Manual of Mental Disorders (5th ed.). Arlington, VA: American Psychiatric Publishing.

Anderson, P. (2002). Assessment and development of executive function (EF) during childhood. *Child Neuropsychology*, 8(2), 71 82.

Aron, A. R., Robbins, T. W., and Poldrack, R. A. (2004). Inhibition and the right inferior frontal cortex. *Trends in Cognitive Sciences*, 8(4), 170-177.

Aron, A., Watkins, L., Sahakian, B., Monsell, S., Barker, R., and Robbins, T. (2003). Task-set switching deficits in early stage Huntington's disease: Implications for basal ganglia function. *Journal of Cognitive Neuroscience*, 15, 629-642.

Avdoshina, V., Bachis, A., and Mocchetti, I. (2013). Synaptic dysfunction in human immunodeficiency virus type-1-positive subjects: inflammation or impaired neuronal plasticity? *Journal of Internal Medicine*, 273, 454-465. doi: 10.1111/joim.12050

Baddeley, A., Bressi, S., Della Sala, S., Logie, R., and Spinnler, H. (1991). The decline of working memory in Alzheimer's disease: A longitudinal study. *Brain,* 114(6), 2521- 2542.

Baddeley, A., Sala, S. D. and Spinnler, H. (1991). The two-component hypothesis of memory deficit in Alzheimer's disease. *Journal of Clinical and Experimental Neuropsychology*, *13*(2), 372-380.

Bagart, B., Camplair, P., and Bourdette, D. (2002). Cognitive dysfunction in Multiple Sclerosis: history, patho-physiology and management. CNS Drugs, 16, 445-55.

Basso, M., Shields, I., Lowery, N., Ghormley, C., Combs, D., Arnett, P., and Johnson, J. (2008). Self-reported executive dysfunction, neuropsychological impairment, functional outcomes in multiple sclerosis. *Journal of Clinical and Experimental Neuropsychology*, 30, 920-930.

Belinger, L., Duff, K., Allison, J., Theriault, D., and O'Rourke, J. (2010). Cognitive change in patients with Huntington's disease on the repeatable battery for the assessment of neuropsychological status. *Journal of Clinical and Experimental Neuropsychology,* 32, 573-578.

Belanger, S., Belleville, S., and Gauthier, S. (2010). Inhibition impairments in Alzheimer's disease, mild cognitive impairment and healthy aging: Effect of congruency proportion in a Stroop task. *Neuropsychologia,* 48(2), 581-590.
doi: 10.1016/j.neuropsychologia.2009.10.021

Best, J. R., Miller, P. H., and Jones, L. L. (2009). Executive functions after age 5: Changes and correlates. *Developmental Review*, 29, 180-200. doi:10.1016 /j.dr.2009.05.002

Blair, C., Raver, C. C., and Berry, D. J. (2014). Two approaches to estimating the effects of parenting on the development of executive function in early childhood. *Developmental Psychology*, 50(2), 554 – 565. doi: 10.1037 /a0033647

Bledsoe, J. C., Semrud-Clikeman, M., and Plizska, S. R. (2013). Anterior cingulate cortex and symptom severity in attention-deficit/hyperactivity disorder. *Journal of Abnormal Psychology,* 122(2), 558-565. doi: 10.1037/a0032390

Bobholz, J., and Rao, S. (2003). Cognitive dysfunction in Multiple Sclerosis: Review of recent developments. *Current Opinions in Neurology*, 16, 283-288.

Bonelli, R. M., and Cummings, J. L. (2007). Frontal-subcortical circuitry and behavior *Dialogues in clinical neuroscience*, 9(2), 141.

Brassington, J., and Marsh, N. (1998). Neuropsychological aspects of Multiple Sclerosis. *Neuropsychology Review*, 8, 43-77.

BrightFocus Foundation (2014). Retrieved July 10, 2014 from http://www.brightfocus.org/alzheimers/livingwith/everydaylife.html

Brown, P., and Marsden, C. D. (1998). What do the basal ganglia do? *The Lancet,* 351(9118), 1801-1804.

Brown, T. M., Ris, M. D., Beebe, D., Ammerman, R. T., Oppenheimer, S. G., Yeates, K. O., and Enrile, B. G. (2008). Factors of biological risk and reserve associated with executive behaviors in children and adolescents with spina bifida myelomeningocele. *Child Neuropsychology*, 14, 118-134. doi: 10.1080/09297040601147605

Bull, R., and Scerif, G. (2001). Executive functioning as a predictor of children's mathematics ability: Inhibition, switching, and working memory. *Developmental neuropsychology*, 19(3), 273-293.

Burmeister, R., Hannay, H. J., Copeland, K., Fletcher, J. M., Boudousquie, A., and Dennis, M. (2005). Attention problems and executive functions in children with spina bifida and hydrocephalus. *Child Neuropsychology*, 11, 265-283. doi: 10.1080/09297049091l324

Burns, A., Jacoby, R., and Levy, R. (1990). Psychiatric phenomena in Alzheimer's disease. IV. Disorders of behavior. *The British Journal of Psychiatry*, 157, 86-94. doi: 10.1192/bjp.157.1.86

Burzynska, A. Z., Nagel, I. E., Preuschhof, C., Gluth, S., Backman, L., Li, S.C., Lindenberger, U., and Heekeren, H. R. (2012). Cortial thickness is linked to executive functioning in adulthood and aging. *Human Brain Mapping*, 33, 1607-1620. doi: 10.1002/hbm.21311

Calabresi, P. Picconi, B., Parnetti, L., and Filippo, M. (2006). A convergent model for cognitive dysfunctions in Parkinson's disease: the critical dopamine- acetylcholine synaptic balance. *Lancet Neurology*, 5, 1-10.

Calderon, J., Perry, R., Erzinclioglu, S., Berrios, G., Dening, R., and Hodges, J. (2001). Perception, attention, and working memory are disproportionately impaired in dementia with Lewy bodies compared to Alzheimer's disease. *Journal of Neurology, Neurosurgery, and Psychiatry*, 70, 157-164. doi:10.1136/jnnp.70.2.157

Carlson, M., Eldreth, D., Chuang, Y., and Eaton, W. (2012). *Public Mental Health* (pp. 253-254). New York, NY: Oxford University Press.

Casari, E. and Fantino, A. (1998). A longitudinal study of cognitive abilities and achievement status of children with myelomeningocele and their relationship with clinical types. *European Journal of Pediatric Surgery*, 8, 152-54.

Castellanos, F. X., Sonuga-Barke, E. J., Milham, M. P., and Tannock, R. (2006). Characterizing cognition in ADHD: beyond executive dysfunction. *Trends in cognitive sciences,* 10(3), 117-123.

Center of Disease Control and Prevention (2012). Monitoring selected national HIV prevention and care objectives by using HIV surveillance data—United States and 6 U.S. dependent areas—2010. *HIV Surveillance Supplemental Report*, 17(3), part A.

Center of Disease Control and Prevention (2013). SpinaBifida. Retreieved March 18, 2014, from http://www.cdc.gov/ncbddd/spinabifida/facts.html

Center of Disease Control and Prevention (2014). HIV/AIDS. Retreieved March 18, 2014, from http://www.cdc.gov/hiv/basics/index.html

Chang, L., Wang, G. J., Volkow, N. D., Ernst, T., Telang, F., Logan, J., and Fowler, J. S. (2004). Decreased brain dopamine transporters are related to cognitive deficits in HIV patients with or without cocaine abuse. *Neuroimage,* 42(2), 869-878.

Chiaravalloti, N.,and DeLuca, J. (2008). Cognitive impairment in Multiple Sclerosis. *Lancet Neurology*, 7, 1139-1151.

Collette F, Van der Linden M, Bechet S, Belleville S, and Salmon, E. (1997). Working memory deficits in Alzheimer's disease. *Brain and Cognition*, 37(1), 147-149.

Conneally, M. (1984). Huntington's Disease: Genetics and Epidemiology. *American Journal of Human Genetics*, 36, 506-526.

Cools, R., Barker, R., Sahakain, B., and Robbins, T. (2001). Mechanisms of cognitive set flexibility in Parkinson's disease. *Brain,* 124, 2563-2512.

Cooper, J., Sagar, H., Tidswell, P and Jordan, N. (1994). Slowed central processing in simple and go/no-go reaction time tasks in Parkinson's disease, *Brain,* 117, 517-529.

Damasio, H., Grabowski, T., Frank, R., Galaburda, A. M., and Damasio, A. R. (1994). The return of Phineas Gage: Clues about the brain from the skull of a famous patient. *Science*, 264(5162), 1102-1105.

Dauer, W. and Przedborski, S. (2003). Parkinson's disease: Mechanisms and models. *Neuron*, 36, 1-10.

Deloire, M., Salort, E., Bonnet, M., Arimone, Y., Boudineau, M., Amieva, H., Barroso, B., Ouallet, J.C., Pachai, C., Galliaud, E., Petry, K.G., Dousset, V., Fabrigoule, C., and Brochet, B. (2005). Cognitive impairment as marker of diffuse brain abnormalities in early relapsing remitting multiple sclerosis. *Journal of Neurology, Neurosurgery, and Psychiatry*, 76, 519-526. doi:10.1136/jnnp.2004.045872

DeLuca, J., Chelune, G., Tulsky, D., Lengenfelder, J., and Chiaravalloti, N. (2004). Is speed of processing or working memory the primary information processing deficit in MS? *Journal of Clinical and Experimental Neuropsychology*, 20, 550-562.

DeLuca., J., and Nocentini, U. (2011). Neuropsychological medical and rehabilitative management of persons with Multiple Sclerosis. *NeuroRehabilitation,* 20, 197-219. DOI: 10.3233/NRE-2011.0695.

Dennis, M. and Barnes, M. A. (2010). The cognitive phenotype of spina bifida meningomyelocele. *Developmental Disabilities*, 16, 31-39. doi: 10.1002 /mrdd.89

Dirnberger, G. and Jahanshahi, M. (2013) Executive dysfunction in Parkinson's disease: A review. *Journal of Neuropsychology*, 7, 193-224.

Dujardin, K., Donze, A., and Hautecoeur, P. (2003). Attention impairment in recently diagnosed multiple sclerosis. *European Journal of Neurology*, 5(1), 61-66. doi: 10.1046/j.1468-1331.1998.510061.x

Eddy, C., Mahalingappa, S., Richards, H. (2012). Is Huntington's disease associated with deficits in theory of mind? *Acta Neurologica Scandinavica*, 126, 376-383. DOI: 10.1111/j.`600-0404.2012.01659.x

Encephalitis Society (2013). HIV-Encephalopathy Information Page. Retrieved on March 31, 2014 from http://www.encephalitis.info/information/types-of-encephalitis/hiv-encephalitis/.

Faiss, J. (2007). Cognitive dysfunction different stages of multiple sclerosis-presentation of 3 cases. *Journal of Neurology*, 254, II/77-II/79. doi: 10.1007/s00415-007-2018-1.

Farinpour, R., Martin, E., Seidenberg, M., Pitrak, D., Pursell, J., Mulane, K., Novak, R.M., and Harrow, M. (2000). Verbal working memory in HIV-seropositive drug users. *Journal of International Neuropsychological Society*, 6, 548-555.

Favre, E., Ballanger, B., Thobois, S., Broussolle, E and Boulinguez, P. (2013). Deep brain Stimulation of the subthalamic nucleus but not dopaminergic medication improves proactive inhibitory control of movement initiation in Parkinson's disease. *Journal of Neurological therapeutics*, 10, 154-167.

Fisk, J. E., and Sharp, C. A. (2004). Age-related impairment in executive functioning: Updating, inhibition, shifting, and access. *Journal of Clinical and Experimental Neuropsychology*, 26(7), 874-890.

Foltynie, J., Brayne, C., Rubbins, T., and Barker, R. (2004). The cognitive ability of an incident cohort of Parkinson's patients in the UK. *Brain*, 127, 550-560.

Foster, P., Drago, V., Yung, R., Cucian, G., and Heilman, K. (2013). Working Memory in Parkinson's Disease: The effects of depression and side of onset of motor symptoms. *Neuropsychology,* 27, 303-313. doi: 10.1037/a0032265.

Fletcher, J. M., Brookshire, B. L., Landry, S. H., Bohan, T. P., Davidson, K. C., Francis, D. J., Leviv, H.S., Harvey, S., Brandt, M.E., Kramer, L.A., and Morris, R. D. (1996). Attentional skills and executive functions in children with early hydrocephalus. *Developmental Neuropsychology*, 12, 53-76. doi:10.1080/ 87565649609540640

Gasquoine, P. G. (2013). Localization and function in anterior cingulate cortex: From psychosurgery to functional neuroimaging. Neuroscience and Biobehavioral Reviews, 37, 340-348. doi: 10.1016/j.neubiorev.2013.01.002

Gilbert, B., Belleville, S., Bherer, L., and Choinard, S. (2005). Study of verbal working memory in patient with Parkinson's disease. *Neuropsychology*, 19(1), 106-114. doi: 10.1037/0894-4105.19.1.106

Gioia, G. and Isquith, P., (2004). Ecological Assessment of Executive Function in Traumatic Brain Injury. *Developmental Neuropsychology*, 25 (1 and 2), 135-158.

Goverover, Y., Chairavalloti, N., and DeLuca, J. (2005). The relationship between self awareness of neurobehavioral symptoms, cognitive functioning and emotional symptoms in multiple sclerosis. *Multiple Sclerosis*, 11, 203-212. DOI: 10.1191/1352458505ms1153.

Grant, I., and Heaton, R. K. (1990). Human immunodeficiency virus-type 1 (HIV-1) and the brain. *Journal of Consulting and Clinical Psychology*, 58, 22-30. doi: 10.1037/0022-006X.58.1.22

Gronning, M., Hannisdal, E., and Mellgren S. (1990). Multivariate analysis of factors associated with unemployment in people with Multiple Sclerosis. *Journal of Neurology, Neurosurgery and Psychiatry*,53, 388-390.

Group, H. (1993). A novel gene containing trinucleotide repeat that is expanded and unstable on Huntington's chromosomes. The Huntington's Disease Collaborative Research Group. *Cell,* 72, 971-983.

Gwinn, M., Pappaioanou, M., George, R., Hannon, W., Wasser, S., Redus, M., Hoff, R., Grady, G.F., Willoughby, A., Novello, A.C., Petersen, L.R., Dondero Jr, T.J., and Curran, J., (1991). Prevalence of HIV infection in childbearing women in the United States: Surveillance using newborn blood samples. *Journal of American Medical Association*, 265(13), 1704-1708. doi:10.1001 /jama.1991.03460130096029

Haaxma, C., Bloem, B., Borm, G., Oyen, W., Leenders, K., Eshuis, S., Boolj, J., Dluzen, D., and Horstink, M. (2007). Gender differences in Parkinson's Disease. *Journal of Neurology, Neurosurgery, Psychiatry*, 78, 819-824.

Hebert, L.E., Weuve, J., Scherr, P.A., and Evans, D.A. (2013). Alzheimer disease in the United States (2010–2050) estimated using the 2010 census. *Neurology,* 80, 1778-1783.

Heffelfinger, A. K., Koop, J. I., Fastenau, P. S., Brei, T. J., Conant, L., Katzenstein, J., Cashin, S.E., and Sawin, K. J. (2008). The relationship of neuro-psychological functioning to adaptation outcome in adolescents with spina bifida. *Journal of the International Neuropsychological Society*, 14(05), 793-804. doi: 10.1017/S1355617708081022

Iddon, J. L., Morgan, D. J. R., Loveday, C., Sahakian, B. J., and Pickard, J. D. (2004). Neuropsychological profile of young adults with spina bifida with or without hydrocephalus. *Journal of Neurology, Neurosurgery and Psychiatry*, 75, 1112-1118. doi: 10.1136/jnnp.2003.029058

Joiner, T. (2009). Why people die by suicide. Harvard University Press. Jonides, J., Schumacher, E. H., Smith, E. E., Lauber, E. J., Awh, E., Minoshima, S., and Koeppe, R. A. (1997). Verbal working memory load affects regional brain activation as measured by PET. *Journal of Cognitive Neuroscience*, 9(4), 462-475.

Kaller, C. P., Rahm, B., Spreer, J., Weiller, C., and Unterrainer, J. M. (2011). Dissociable contributions of left and right dorsolateral prefrontal cortex in planning. *Cerebral Cortex,* 21, 307-317. doi:10.1093/cercor/bhq096

Kelly, N. C., Ammerman, R. T., Rausch, J. R., Ris, M. D., Yeates, K. O., Oppenheimer, S. G., and Enrile, B. G. (2012). Executive functioning and psychological adjustment in children and youth with spina bifida. *Child Neuropsychology,* 18, 417-431. doi: 10.1080/09297049.2011.613814

King, A., Valenca, A., de Oliveira e Silva, A., Cerqueira, A., Ferraz, L., and Nardi, A. (2011). Huntington's disease: Two-year observational follow-up of executive function evaluation with CNS vital signs test in an adult patient. *Case Reports in Medicine*, 1-5. DOI: 10.1155/2011/380894.

Klempir, J., Klempirova, O., Stochl, J., Spachova, N., and Roth, J. (2009). The relationship between impairment of voluntary movements and cognitive impairment in Huntington's disease. *Journal of Neurology*, 256, 1629-1633. DOI: 10.1007/s00415-009-5164-9.

Koekkoek, S., de Sonneville, L., Wolfs, T., Licht, R., and Geelen, S. (2008). Neurocognitive function profile in HIV-infected school-age children. European *Journal of Paediatric Neurology*, 12(4), 290-297.

doi:http://dx.doi.org/10.1016/j.ejpn.2007.09.002

Kornblith, A., LaRocca, N., and Baum, H. (1986). Employment in inidividuals with multiple Sclerosis. *International Journal of Rehabilitative Research*, 9, 155-165.

Krause, I., Kern, S., Horntrich, A., and Ziemssen, T. (2013). Employment status in multiple sclerosis: Impact of disease specific and non disease specific factors. Multiple Sclerosis Journal, 19, 1792-1799. DOI: 10.1177/1352458513485655.

Kudlicka, A., Clare, L., and Hindle, J. (2011). Quality of life, health status, and caregiver burden in Parkinson's disease: Relationship to executive functioning. *Journal of Geriatric Psychology*, 29. 68-76. DOI: 10.1002/gps.3970

Kurtzke, J. (2000). Multiple Sclerosis in time and space- geographic clues to cause. *Journal of Neurovirology*, 6, S134-S140.

Landry, K., and Smith, T. (1998). Neurocognitive effects of HIV infection on young children implications for assessment. *Topics in Early Childhood Special Education,* 18, 160-169.

Laughton, B., Cornell, M., Boivin, M., and Rie, A. V. (2013). Neurodevelopment in perinatally HIV-infected children: A concern for adolescence. *Journal of the International AIDS Society,* 16, 1-11. doi: 10.7448/IAS.16.1.18603

Lawrence, A., Sahakian, B., Hodges, J., Roseer, A., Lange, K., and Robbins, T. (1996). Executive and mnemonic functions in early Huntington's disease. *Brain,* 119, 1633-1645.

Lawrence, A., Sahakian, B., and Robbins, T. (1998). Cognitive functions and corticostriatal circuits: insights from Huntington's Disease. *Trends in Cognitive Science,* 2, 1-10.

Lawson, G. M., Duda, J. T., Avants, B. B., Wu, J., and Farah, M. (2013). Associations between children's socioeconomic status and prefrontal cortical thickness. *Developmental Science*, 16(5), 641-652. doi: 10.1111/desc.12096

Mammarella, N., Cornoldi, C., and Donadello, E. (2003). Visual but not spatial working memory deficit in children with spina bifida. *Brain and Cognition*, 53(2), 311-314. doi: 10.1016/S0278-2626(03)00132-5

Minassian, A., Henry, B., Woods, S., Vaida, F., Grant, I., Geyer, M., and Perry, W. (2013). Prepulse inhibition in HIV-associated neurocognitive disorders. *Journal of the International Neuropsychological Society*, 19(6), 709-717.

Mitchell, W. (2001). Neurological and developmental effects of HIV and AIDS in children and adolescents. Mental Retardation and Developmental Disabilities *Research Reviews*, 7, 211-216. doi: 10.1002/mrdd.1029

Miyake, A., Friedman, N. P., Emerson, M. J., Witzki, A. H., and Howerter, A. (2000). The unity and diversity of executive functions and their contributions to complex "frontal lobe" tasks: A latent variable analysis. *Cognitive Psychology*, 41, 49-100. doi:10.1006/cogp.1999.0734

Monsell, S. (2003). Task switching. *Trends in Cognitive Sciences*, 7(3), 134-140. doi:10.1016/S1364-6613(03)00028-7

Montoya, A., Price, B., Menear, M., and Lepage, M. (2006). Brain imaging and cognitive dysfunctions in Huntington's disease. *Journal of Psychiatry Neuroscience*, 31, 21-29.

Moran, L., Booze, R., and Mactutus, C. (2014). Modeling deficits in attention, inhibition, and flexibility in HAND. *Journal of Neuroimmune Pharmacology*.
doi: 10.1007/s11481-014-9539

Morgan, A. B., and Lilienfeld, S. O., (2000). A meta-analytic review of the relation between antisocial behavior and neuropsychological measures of executive function. *Clinical Psychology Review*, 20(1), 113-136.

Motl, R.W., Arnett, P.A., Smith, M.M., Barwick, F.H., Ahlstrom, B., and Stover, E.J. (2009). Worsening of symptoms is associated with lower physical activity levels in individuals with multiple sclerosis. *Multiple Sclerosis* (13524585), 14(1), 140-142.

Muslimovic, D., Post, B., Spelman, J., and Schmand, B. (2005). Cognitive profile of newly diagnosed people with Parkinson's. *Journal of Neurology*, 65, 1239-1245. DOI: 10.1212/01. Wni.0000120516.69332.45

Nocera, J., Price, C., Fernandez, H., Amano, S., Vallabhajosula, S., Okun, M, Hwynn, N., and Hass, C.J. (2010). Tests of dorsolateral frontal function correlate with objective stability in early to moderate stage Parkinson's disease. *Parkinsonism and Related Disorders*, 16, 590-594.

Novak, M., and Tabrizi, S. (2010). Huntington's disease. *BMJ*, 340, 34-40. doi:10.1136/ bmj.c3109.

Obeso, I., Casabona, E., Bringas, M., Alvarez, L., and Jahanshahi, M. (2012). Semantic and phonemic verbal fluency in Parkinson's disease: Influence of clinical and demographic variables. *Behavioral Neurology*, 25, 111-118. DOI: 10.3233/BEN-2011-0354

Owen, A., James, M., Leigh, P., Summars, B., Marsden, C., Quinn, N.., Lange, K.W., and Robbins, T.W. (1992). Fronto-striatal cognitive deficits at different stages of Parkinson's disease. *Brain*, 115, 1727-1751.

Parker, K., Lamichhane, D., Caetao, M., and Narayanan, N. (2013). Executive dysfunction in Parkinson's disease and timing deficits. Frontiers in Integrative *Neuroscience,* 7, 1-9. doi: 10.3389/fnint.2013.0075

Perry, R., and Hodges, J. (1998). Attention and executive deficits in Alzheimer's disease: A critical review. *The Journals of Gerontology: Series B,* 52B(1), 28-39.

Pierson, S., and Griffith, N. (2006). Treatment of cognitive impairment in Multiple Sclerosis. *Behavioral Neurology*, 17, 53-67.

Price, R. W., Brew, B., Sidtis, J., Rosenblum, M., Scheck, A. C., and Cleary, P. (1988). The brain in AIDS: central nervous system HIV-1 infection and AIDS dementia complex. *Science,* 239, 586-592. doi: 10.1126/science.3277272

Raichle, M. E. (1994). Images of the mind: Studies with modern imaging techniques. *Annual Review of Psychology*, 45, 33-356. doi: 10.1146/annurev. ps.45.020194.002001

Reingold, S. (1995). *Research directions in Multiple Sclerosis*. New York. USA: National Multiple Sclerosis Society.

de Rijk, M., Launer, L., Berger, K., Breteler, M., Dartigues, J., Baldereschi, M., Fratiglioni, L., Lobo, A., Martinez-Lage, J., Trenkwalder, C., and Hofman, A. (2000). Prevalence of Parkinson's disease in Europe: A collaborative study of population based cohorts. *Neurology,* 54, 21-23.

Rogalsky, C., Vidal, C., Li, X., and Damasio, H. (2012). Risky decision-making in older adults without cognitive deficits: An fMRI study of VMPFC using the Iowa Gambling Task. *Social Neuroscience*, 7(2), 178-190. doi: 10.1080/17470919.2011.588340

Roos, R., Hermans, J., Vegter-van der Vlis, M., van Ommen, G., and Bruyn, G., (1993). Duration of illness in Huntington's disease is not related to age at onset. *Journal of Neurology, Neurosurgery and Psychiatry*, 56, 98-100.

Rose, B. M., and Holmbeck, G. N. (2007). Attention and executive functions in adolescents with spina bifida. *Journal of Pediatric Psychology*, 32, 983-994. doi: 10.1093/jpepsy/jsm042

Ross, R. S., LoPresti, M. L., Schon, K., and Chantal, E. S. (2013). Role of the hippocampus and orbitofrontal cortex during the disambiguation of social cues in working memory. *Cognitive, Affective, and Behavioral Neuroscience*, 13, 900-915. doi: 10.3758/s13415-013-0170-x

Ruscheweyh, R., Deppe, M., Lohmann, H., Wersching, H., Korsukewitz, C., Duning, T., Bluhm, S., Stehling, C., Keller, S.S., and Knecht, S. (2013). Executive performance is related to regional gray matter volume in healthy older individuals. *Human Brain Mapping*, 34, 3333-3346. doi: 10.1002/hbm.22146

Salthouse, T. A. (2005). Relations between cognitive abilities and measures of executive functioning. *Neuropsychology*, 19(4), 532.

Salthouse, T. A., Atkinson, T. M. and Berish, D. E. (2003). Executive functioning as a potential mediator of age-related cognitive decline in normal adults. *Journal of Experimental Psychology: General*, *132*(4), 566.

Salthouse, T. A., Fristoe, N., McGuthry, K. E. and Hambrick, D. Z. (1998). Relation of task switching to speed, age, and fluid intelligence. *Psychology and aging*, *13*(3), 445.

Schon, K., Ross, R. S., Hasselmo, M. E., and Stern, C. E. (2013). Complementary roles of medial temporal lobes and mid-dorsolateral prefrontal cortex for working memory for novel and familiar trial-unique visual stimuli. European *Journal of Neuroscience*, 37, 668-678. doi:10.1111/ejn.12062

Schnitzspahn, K. M., Stahl, C., Zeintl, M., Kaller, C. P., and Kliegel, M. (2013). The role of shifting, updating, and inhibition in prospective memory performance in young and older adults. *Developmental Psychology*, 49(8), 1544.

Shelton, J., Elliot, E., Hill, B.D., Calamia, M., and Gouvier, D. (2011). A comparison of laboratory and clinical working memory tests and their prediction of fluid intelligence. *Intelligence,* 37283-293. doi:10.1016 /j.intell.2008.11.005

Simpson, D. M., and Tagliati, M. (1994). Neurologic manifestations of HIV infection. *Annals of Internal Medicine*, 121, 769-785. doi: 10.7326/0003-4819-121-10-199411150-00008

Sitek, E., Soltan, W., Wieczorek, D., Schinwelski, M., Robowski, P., Harciarek, M., Guzińska, K., and Sławek, J. (2013). Self-awareness of executive dysfunction in Huntington's disease: Comparison with Parkinson's disease and cervical dystonia. *Psychiatry and Clinical Neurosciences*, 67, 59-62. doi: 10.1111/pcn.12006

Smith, M., and Arnett, P. (2010). Awareness of executive functioning deficits in multiple sclerosis: Self-versus informant ratings of impairment. *Journal of Clinical and Experimental Neuropsychology*, 32, 780-787. DOI: 10.1080 /13803390903543O7.

Snow, J. H., Prince, M., Souheaver, G., Ashcraft, E., Stefans, V., and Edmonds, J. (1994). Neuropsychological patterns of adolescents and young adults with spina bifida. *Archives of Clinical Neuropsychology*, 9(3), 277-287.

Soare, P. L., and Raimondi, A. J. (1977). Intellectual and perceptual-motor characteristics of treated myelomeningocele children. *Archives of Pediatrics and Adolescent Medicine*, 131, 199-204. doi: 10.1001/archpedi.1977. 02120150081017.

Spina Bifida Association of America (2014). "A Guide for Medical Professionals." Retrieved on March 31, 2014 from http://www.spinabifidaassociation.org/site/c.evKRI7OXIoJ8H/b.8340105/k.2BC8/A_Gui de_For_Medical_Professionals.htm.

Sprengelmeyer, R., Young, A., Calder, A., Karrat, A., Lange, H., Hömberg, V., Perrett, D..I, and Rowland, D. (1996). Loss of disgust: Perception of faces and emotions in Huntington's Disease, *Brain*, 119, 1647-1665.

Staples, D., Lincoln, N. (1979). Intellectual impairment and its relation to functional abilities. *Rheumatology Rehabilitation*, 18, 153-160.

Stout, J., Salmon, D., Butters, N., Taylor, M., Peavy, G., Heindel, W., Delis, D.C., Ryan, L., Atkinson, J.H., Chandler, J.L., Grant, I., and the HNRC Group. (1995). Decline in working memory associated with HIV infection. *Psychological Medicine*, 25, 1221-1232. doi:10.1136/jnnp.2004.045872

Stubberud, J. and Riemer, G. (2012). Problematic psychosocial adaptation and executive dysfunction in women and men with myelomeningocele. *Disability and Rehabilitation*, 34, 740-746. doi: 10.3109/09638288.2011.619617

Suchy, Y. (2009). Executive functioning: Overview, assessment, and research issues for non-neuropsychologists. *Annual Behavioral Medicine*, 37, 106-116. doi: 10.1007/s12160-009-9097-4

Suhr, J. (1997). Executive functioning deficits in hypothetically psychosis-prone college students. *Schizophrenia Research* 27, 29-35.

Sylvester, C. Y. C., Wager, T. D., Lacey, S. C., Hernandez, L., Nichols, T. E., Smith, E. E., and Jonides, J. (2003). Switching attention and resolving interference: fMRI measures of executive functions. *Neuropsychologia*, 41(3), 357-370.

Takeuchi, H., Taki, Y., Sassa, Y., Hashizume, H., Sekiguchi, A., Fukushima, A., and Kawashima, R. (2013). *Brain Structure and Function*, 218, 1017-1032. doi: 10.1007/s00429-012-0444-z

Tannock, R. (1998). Attention deficit hyperactivity disorder: advances in cognitive, neurobiological, and genetic research. *Journal of Child Psychology and Psychiatry,* 39(1), 65-99.

Tuminello, E. R., Holmbeck, G. N., and Olson, R. (2012). Executive functions in adolescents with spina bifida: Relations with autonomy development and parental intrusiveness. *Child Neuropsychology*, 18, 105-124. doi: 10.1080 /09297049.2011.590470

Vance, D. E., Fazeli, P. L., Moneyham, L., Keltner, N. L., and Raper, J. L. (2013). Assessing and treating forgetfulness and cognitive problems in adults with HIV. *Journal of the Association of Nurses in AIDS Care,* 24, S40-S60. doi: 10.1016/j.jana.2012.03.006

Van Den Eeden, S., Tanner, C., Berstein, A., Fross, R., Leimpeter, A., Bloch, D., and Nelson, L. (2002). Incidence of Parkinson's disease: variation by age, gender, race/ethnicity. *American Journal of Epidemiology*, 157, 1015-1022.

van der Ven, S. H. G., Kroesbergen, E. H., Boom, J., and Leseman, P. P. M. (2013). The structure of executive functions in children: A closer examination of inhibition, shifting, and updating. *British Journal of Developmental Psychology*, 31, 70-87. doi: 10.1111/j.2044-835X.2012.02079.x

Weintraub, D., Comella, C., and Horn, S. (2008). Parkinson's disease part 1: Pathophysiology, symptoms, burden, diagnosis and assessment. *American Journal of Managed Care*, 14, 40-48.

Weintraub, S., Wicklund, A.H., and Salmon, D., (2012). The Neuropsychological Profile of Alzheimer Disease. *Cold Spring Harbor Perspectives in Medicine*, 2:a006171

Willcutt, E. G., Doyle, A. E., Nigg, J. T., Faraone, S. V., and Pennington, B. F. (2005). Validity of the executive function theory of attention-deficit /hyperactivity disorder: a meta-analytic review. *Biological Psychiatry*, 57(11), 1336-1346.

Williams, L.J., Mai, C., Edmonds, L., Shaw, G., Kirby, R., Hobbs, C., Sever, L.E., Miller, L.A., Meaney, F.J., and Levitt, M. (2002). Prevalence of spina bifida and anencephaly during the transition to mandatory folic acid fortification in the United States. *Teratology,* 66(1), 33-39.

Williams, L., Rasmussen, S., Flores, A., Kirby, R., and Edmonds, L. (2005). Decline in the prevalence of spina bifida and anencephaly by race/ethnicity: 1995-2002. *Pediatrics* 116(3), 580-586. doi: 10.1542/peds.2005-0592

Williams-Gray, C., Evans, J., Gons, A., Foltynie, T., Ban, M., Robbins, T., Brayne, C., Kolachana, B., Wenberger, D., Sawcer, S., Barker, R. (2009). The Distinct cognitive syndromes of Parkinson's disease: 5 year follow up of the campaign cohort. *Brain*, 132, 2958-2989. doi: 10.1093/brain/awp345

Willis, M. L., Palermo, R., McGrillen, K., and Miller, L. (2014). The nature of facial expression recognition deficits following orbitofrontal cortex damage. *Neuropsychology,* 1, 1-11. doi: 10.1037/neu0000059

Wills, K. W. (1993). Neuropsychological functioning in children with spina bifida and/or hydrocephalus. *Journal of Clinical Child Psychology*, 22, 247-265. doi: 10.1207/s15374424jccp2202_11

Wills, K. E., Holmbeck, G. N., Dillon, K., and McLone, D. G. (1988). Intelligence and achievement in children with myelomeningocele. *Journal of Pediatric Psychology,* 15, 161-176. doi: 10.1093/jpepsy/15.2.161

Woods, S. P., Moore, D. J., Weber, E., and Grant, I. (2009). Cognitive neuropsychology of HIV-associated neurocognitive disorders. *Neuropsychology Review*, 19, 152-168. doi: 10.1007/s11065-009-9102-5

Wylie, S., Wildenberg, W., Ridderinkhof, K., Classen, D., Wooten, G., Manning, C. (2012). Differential susceptibility to motor impulsivity among functional subtypes of Parkinson's disease. *Journal of Neurology, Neurosurgery and Psychiatry,* 83, 1149-1154. doi: 10.1136/jnnp-2012-303056.

Zachary, R. B. (1977). Life with spina bifida. *British Medical Journal*, 2(6100), 1460.

Zelazo, P. D., and Carlson, S. M. (2012). Hot and cool executive function in childhood and adolescence: Development and plasticity. *Child Development Perspectives,* 6(4), 354-360. doi: 10.1111/j.1750-8606.2012.00246.x

In: Research Trends in Behavior …
Editor: Miao-Kun Sun
ISBN: 978-1-63485-461-0

Chapter 2

ROLE OF LONG-CHAIN OMEGA-3 FATTY ACIDS IN CORTICAL CIRCUIT MATURATION: IMPLICATIONS FOR PSYCHOPATHOLOGY

Robert K. McNamara**, Ph.D.
Department of Psychiatry and Behavioral Neuroscience,
University of Cincinnati College of Medicine, Cincinnati US

ABSTRACT

Increasing translational evidence suggests that long-chain omega-3 (LC*n*-3) fatty acids, including eicosapentaenoic acid (EPA, 20:5*n*-3) and docosahexaenoic acid (DHA, 22:6*n*-3), play a critical role in brain development. DHA has anti-inflammatory, neurotrophic, and neuroprotective properties and accumulates in the brain during active periods of perinatal cortical expansion and functional connectivity. Rodent studies demonstrate that reductions in perinatal rat brain DHA accrual are associated with delays in neuronal migration and arborization, synaptic pathology, neurocognitive deficits, and elevated behavioral indices of aggression and depression. Non-human primates raised on an *n*-3 fatty acid deficient diet exhibit hyperactivity, impairments in visual

* Correspondence and requests for reprints: Robert K. McNamara, Ph.D., Department of Psychiatry and Behavioral Neuroscience, University of Cincinnati College of Medicine, 260 Stetson Street, Cincinnati, OH 45219-0516 PH: 513-558-5601 FAX: 513-558-4805 E-mail: robert.mcnamara@uc.edu

attention, and functional connectivity deficits within cortical networks. Human preterm delivery is associated with early deficits in cortical DHA accrual, enduring reductions in cortical circuit connectivity, and increased risk for developing psychiatric disorders including unipolar depression, bipolar disorder, and schizophrenia. These psychiatric disorders commonly initially emerge during adolescence, a developmental period associated with rapid and dynamic changes cortical circuit maturation, and are associated with LC*n*-3 fatty acid deficits. This body of translational evidence suggests that deficits in LC*n*-3 fatty acids during perinatal development may contribute to impaired cortical circuit maturation and associated risk for psychiatric disorders. Developing a more comprehensive understanding of the requirement for LC*n*-3 fatty acids during normal human perinatal brain development could therefore have significant implications for informing optimal intake levels during critical periods of neurodevelopment.

Keywords: Omega-3 fatty acids, Docosahexaenoic acid (DHA), Brain development, Attention deficit/hyperactivity disorder (ADHD), Mood, Cognition, Bipolar disorder, Schizophrenia; Prefrontal cortex, Amygdala.

1. Introduction

Major psychiatric disorders including major depressive disorder (MDD), bipolar disorder, schizophrenia, and attention deficit hyperactivity disorder (ADHD) are prominent causes of premature disability and mortality. In the United States (U.S.), severe forms of MDD currently affect between 2-7%, and up to 16-20% suffer from milder forms of the illness, and life-time prevalence estimates for bipolar disorder are 1.0% for bipolar-I, 1.1% for bipolar-II, and 2.4% for subthreshold bipolar disorder (4.4% total)(Kessler et al., 2007). Bipolar disorder is commonly preceded by several years of attenuated mood symptoms and neurocognitive impairment particularly in concentration/attention (Conus et al., 2008; McNamara et al., 2010a). In the U.S., ADHD is the most common childhood psychiatric disorder with prevalence rates ranging from 5-16% (Polanczyk et al., 2007), and schizophrenia has a life-time prevalence rate of approximately 1.0% (McGuffin et al., 2004). Mood and psychotic disorders are chronic and typically recurring illnesses associated with excess premature mortality attributable primarily to suicide and cardiovascular-related diseases (Angst et al., 2002; Brown et al., 1997; Osby et al., 2001). These disorders also have a significant economic impact due in part to excess health care utilization and lost productivity (Greenberg et al., 2003; Kleinman et al., 2003; Meyers et al., 2010; Wu et al., 2005). Psychiatric symptoms typically require long-term treatment with pharmacological agents and symptomatic relapse following medication discontinuation is common (Ayuso-Gutierrez and del Rio Vega, 1997; Cavanagh et al., 2004; Geddes et al., 2003). Therefore, developing a better understanding of the risk and resilience mechanisms associated with the initial development of psychopathology represents an urgent public health need.

The pathogenic mechanisms underlying major psychiatric disorders are viewed as polygenic and multifactorial. Indeed, subtotal heritability estimates and monozygotic twin discordance rates indicate that both genetic and environmental factors confer vulnerability and offspring of first degree relatives with mood or psychotic disorders have an elevated risk of developing psychiatric disorders (Ehringer et al., 2006; Sullivan et al., 2000; Tsuang et al., 2000). An important clue into the pathoetiology of psychiatric disorders may come from when they initially emerge during the lifespan. The initial onset of major mood and psychotic disorders frequently occur during adolescence or early adulthood (Burke et al., 1991; Kessler et al., 2005; Perlis et al., 2009), a developmental period associated with rapid and dynamic changes in prefrontal cortex (PFC) structural maturation in typically developing youth (Geidd et al., 2009). Specifically, the period between childhood and early adolescence (7-12 years) is associated with the rapid expansion of gray matter density in the PFC, and the period between adolescence (13-18 years) and young adulthood (≥18 years) is associated with a progressive loss of cortical gray matter density and reciprocal increases in white matter density in fronto-limbic fiber tracts (Geidd et al., 2009). Consistent with a neurodevelopmental etiology, converging evidence from cross-sectional and longitudinal structural magnetic resonance imaging (MRI) studies have found that psychiatric disorders are associated with deficits in PFC functional integrity and associated abnormalities in connectivity with limbic and striatal structures (reviewed below). Therefore, the initial onset of major psychiatric disorders coincides with active and dynamic changes in PFC structural maturation, and perturbations in these maturational processes may contribute to the later emergence of psychopathology.

While the risk and resilience mechanisms associated with abnormal PFC circuit development in psychiatric disorders are not known, a substantial body of evidence has emerged over the last twenty years which suggest that psychiatric disorders including MDD, bipolar disorder, schizophrenia, and ADHD are associated with deficits in long-chain omega-3 (LC*n*-3) fatty acids. Moreover, emerging evidence from preclinical studies and preliminary human MRI studies suggest that LC*n*-3 fatty acid deficiency during perinatal development directly impacts PFC structural and functional connectivity. The objective of this review is to critically evaluate translational evidence implicating LC*n*-3 fatty acids in PFC development and explore the potential role of LC*n*-3 fatty acid deficiency in the PFC circuit maturation deficits observed in psychiatric disorders.

2. LC*N*-3 FATTY ACID DEFICIENCY AND PSYCHIATRIC DISORDERS

As background, mammals require a dietary source of *n*-3 fatty acids to procure and maintain adequate concentrations of LC*n*-3 fatty acids in peripheral and central tissues. Principle dietary sources of the vegetable short-chain *n*-3 fatty acid precursor α-linolenic acid (ALA, 18:3*n*-3) include flaxseed, linseed, canola, soy, and perilla oils. The biosynthesis of LC*n*-3 fatty acids, including eicosapentaenoic acid (EPA, 20:5*n*-3) and docosahexaenoic acid (DHA, 22:6*n*-3), from ALA requires a series of microsomal reactions mediated by desaturase and elongase enzymes/genes. The rate-limiting enzymes regulating LC*n*-3 fatty acid biosynthesis include delta-6 desaturase (Δ6-desaturase, *FADS2*) and delta-5 desaturase (Δ5-desaturase, *FADS1*), and emerging evidence from human genotyping studies suggest that single nucleotide polymorphisms within *FADS2* and/or *FASD1* genes are an important determinant of LC*n*-3 fatty acid status (Koletzko et al., 2011; Rzehak et al., 2009). The final synthesis of DHA requires β-oxidation within peroxisomes, and heritable polymorphisms in peroxisomal genes are associated with peripheral and central DHA deficits and neuodevelopmental perturbations (Martinez et al., 1992).

In healthy subjects residing in western countries, ALA→EPA biosynthesis is limited and ALA→DHA and EPA→DHA biosynthesis is negligible (Brenna et al., 2009). However, preformed EPA and DHA can be obtained directly from the diet, particularly from fatty cold water fish, including salmon, trout, tuna, as well as fish oil (FO) and algal-derived LC*n*-3 fatty acid supplements. Bypassing microsomal- and peroxisomal-mediated biosynthesis with preformed DHA is significantly more effective than ALA for increasing

DHA composition in erythrocyte (red blood cell) membranes (Barceló-Coblijn et al., 2008), breast milk (Francois ct al., 2003; Jensen et al., 2000) and cortical gray matter (Lin et al., 2011a; Su et al., 1999). Peripheral and central LC*n*-3 fatty acid status is therefore governed by gene-diet interactions.

An individual's LC*n*-3 fatty acid status can be determined using the fatty acid composition of erythrocyte membranes by gas chromatography, and erythrocyte LC*n*-3 fatty acid levels are a valid index of habitual dietary LC*n*-3 fatty acid intake (Fekete et al., 2009). For example, controlled LC*n*-3 fatty acid intervention studies have found that FO supplementation dose-dependently increases erythrocyte LC*n*-3 fatty acid levels in human subjects (Barceló-Coblijn et al., 2008; Flock et al., 2013). Moreover, the greater annual fish and seafood consumption in Japan (148 lb/person) compared with the U.S. (48 lb/person)(WHO, 1996) is associated with a ~2-fold greater erythrocyte membrane EPA+DHA composition in healthy Japanese adults (8.5±1.8%)(Itomura et al., 2008) compared with healthy U.S. adults (4.9±2.1%)(Sands et al., 2005). It is relevant therefore that cross-national epidemiological studies have found that higher per capita intake of fish/seafood is associated with lower lifetime prevalence rates of unipolar and bipolar depression (Hibbeln, 1998, Noaghiul and Hibbeln, 2003; Peet, 2004). Moreover, population studies have found that lower LC*n*-3 fatty acid intake is associated with increased risk for developing depressive symptoms (Astorg et al., 2008; Colangelo et al., 2009; Murakami et al., 2010; Raeder et al., 2007; Tanskanen et al., 2001; Timonen et al., 2004). Together, these data suggest that lower habitual dietary LC*n*-3 fatty acid intake and status may be associated with increased risk for mood dysregulation.

Several independent studies from different countries have observed significant erythrocyte membrane LC*n*-3 fatty acid deficits in MDD patients compared with healthy controls. A recent meta-analysis of 14 case-control studies found significantly lower erythrocyte EPA and DHA levels in MDD patients (Lin et al., 2010). In bipolar patients, three independent studies have observed significant erythrocyte LC*n*-3 fatty acid deficits compared with healthy controls (Chiu et al., 2003; McNamara et al., 2010b; Ranjekar et al., 2003). Importantly, erythrocyte LC*n*-3 fatty acid deficits have also been observed in pediatric and adolescent patients with MDD or bipolar disorder proximal to illness onset (Clayton et al., 2008; Pottala et al., 2012; McNamara et al., 2014). Prospective surveillance studies have found that low baseline LC*n*-3 fatty acid status is a predictor of suicide in MDD patients (Sublette et al., 2006) as well as treatment-emergent depression in human subjects receiving interferon-α (Lotrich et al., 2013; Su et al., 2010). Medication-naïve first-episode psychotic patients exhibit erythrocyte DHA deficits compared with healthy controls (Khan et al., 2002; Reddy et al., 2004), and a recent meta-analysis of 18 case-control studies observed significant DHA deficits in schizophrenic patients (Hoen et al., 2013). A recent meta-analysis of nine cross-sectional studies observed significantly lower blood DHA levels in ADHD children compared with healthy controls (Hawkey and Nigg, 2014). Together, these case-control studies provide evidence that different psychiatric disorders are characterized by low LC*n*-3 fatty acid status which coincide with, and may precede, the initial onset of psychopathology.

The principal LC*n*-3 fatty acid found in mammalian brain gray matter is DHA, which comprises approximately 10-20% of total fatty acid composition in the adult PFC (Carver et al., 2001; Connor et al., 1990; McNamara et al., 2008a). Although the omega-3 fatty acid precursors of DHA, including α-linolenic acid (ALA, 18:3*n*-3), EPA (20:5*n*-3), and docosapentaenoic acid (22:5*n*-3), cross the blood-brain barrier, they are rapidly oxidized and consequently comprise <1% of total brain fatty acid composition (Chen et al., 2009). Erythrocyte and PFC DHA levels are positively correlated under steady state dietary conditions (Carver et al., 2001; Connor et al., 1990), though erythrocyte DHA levels change more rapidly than PFC levels in response to changes in dietary LC*n*-3 fatty acid intake. For example, dietary *n*-3 fatty acid intake during adolescence is an important determinant of rat PFC and erythrocyte DHA levels which are positively correlated in young adulthood (Figure 1). A growing number of case-control studies have investigated the fatty acid composition of postmortem frontal gray matter from patients with mood and psychotic disorders. Some studies have observed lower LC*n*-3 fatty acid levels (McNamara et al., 2007a, 2007b, 2008b; Tatebayashi et al., 2013; Conklin et al., 2010) while others have not (Igarashi et al., 2010; Lalovic et al., 2007; Yao et al., 2000). Our group reported that young adult patients with MDD (McNamara et al., 2007a), bipolar disorder (McNamara et al., 2008a), and schizophrenia (McNamara et al., 2007b) exhibit significant PFC DHA deficits compared with controls. In a preliminary postmortem study, we also found that DHA composition increases sharply in the PFC during normal human adolescent development, and that this increase is significantly blunted in young adult suicide victims (Figure 2). While these findings suggest that psychopathology may be associated with deficits in PFC DHA accrual, limitations associated with the postmortem approach constrain interpretation (McNamara and Jandacek, 2011).

While the etiology of LC*n*-3 fatty acid deficits observed in psychiatric patients is likely multifactorial (McNamara, 2013a), dietary LC*n*-3 fatty acid supplementation has been found to significantly increase patient erythrocyte LC*n*-3 fatty acid levels (Amminger et al., 2010; Clayton et al., 2009; Wozniak et al., 2007). This observation indicates that LC*n*-3 fatty acid deficits in psychiatric patients are modifiable by increasing dietary LC*n*-3 fatty acid intake. Importantly, meta-analyses of controlled trials have observed a significant advantage of LC*n*-3 fatty acid supplementation over placebo for reducing depressive symptoms in patients with MDD (Grosso et al., 2014) or bipolar disorder (Sarris et al., 2012). Preliminary trials have found that LC*n*-3 fatty acid supplementation significantly reduces depression and manic symptom severity in pediatric and adolescent patients (Clayton et al., 2009; McNamara et al., 2014; Nemets et al., 2006; Wozniak et al., 2007). Accumulating evidence also suggests that LC*n*-3 fatty acid supplementation may be efficacious for the treatment of positive and negative symptoms in patients with or at ultra-high risk for developing schizophrenia (Amminger et al., 2010; Emsley et al., 2002; Mellor et al., 1995; Peet et al., 2001), and for reducing attention deficits in pediatric and adolescent ADHD patients (Bloch and Qawasmi, 2011; Hawkey and Nigg, 2014; Vaisman et al., 2008).

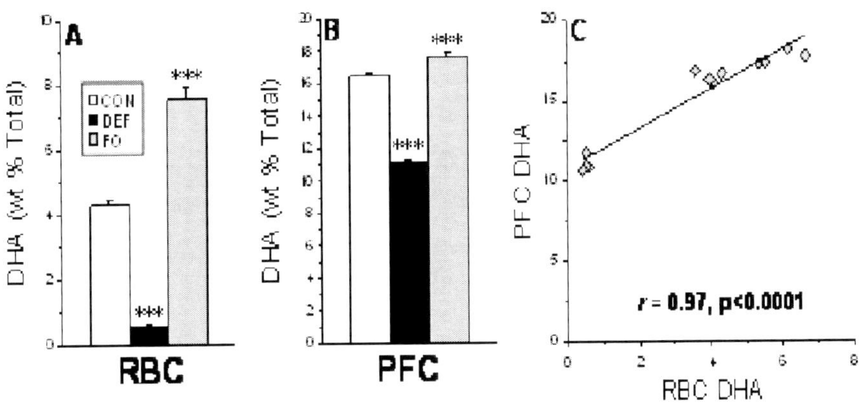

Figure 1. Adult erythrocyte (A) and PFC (B) DHA levels (weight % total fatty acids) in rats fed a control diet (CON) containing 4.9% ALA, a diet containing no *n*-3 fatty acids (DEF), or a diet fortified with fish oil (FO) containing LC*n*-3 fatty acids (2.2% EPA, 1.7% DHA) during peri-adolescent development (postnatal day 21-90). Dietary *n*-3 fatty acid depletion is associated with significant erythrocyte and PFC DHA deficits in young adulthood, and that fortifying the diet with LC*n*-3 fatty acids is associated with significantly greater increases in erythrocyte and PFC DHA levels in young adulthood compared with CON rats. Note that among all rats erythrocyte and PFC DHA levels are positively correlated (C). Values are group means ± S.E.M. ***$p \leq 0.0001$ vs. Controls.

While this body of evidence suggests that low LC*n*-3 fatty acid intake and status may represent a modifiable risk factor for psychopathology, the central mechanisms mediating this relationship remain poorly understood. Over the past 30 years evidence has emerged from both animal and clinical research that suggests that normal brain development requires optimal DHA levels. The following sections provide an overview of evidence from rodent, non-human primate, and human studies investigating the role of LC*n*-3 fatty acids in normal brain development. We then review evidence from neuroimaging studies implicating low LC*n*-3 fatty acid intake and status in cortical circuit maturation impairments observed in psychiatric disorders.

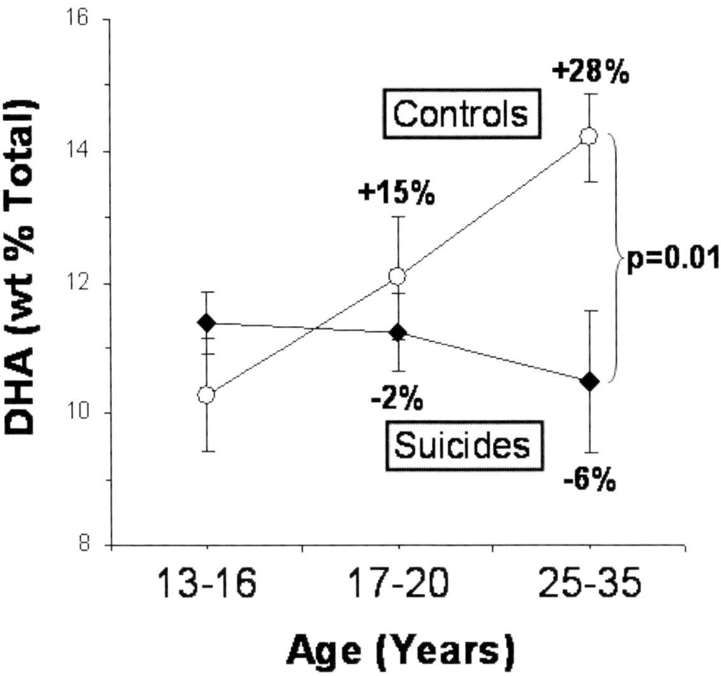

Figure 2. Comparison of DHA levels (weight % total fatty acids) in the human postmortem PFC (BA10) of typically developing adolescents and young adults and suicide victims (n=8-12/age group). Note that DHA levels progressively increase in the PFC of typically developing adolescents but not in suicide victims. Values are group means ± S.E.M.

3. Rodent Neurodevelopment

In rodents unesterified DHA diffuses from plasma to brain at a rate that is equilibrated with brain DHA consumption (Ouellet et al., 2009; Rapoport et al., 2011), and preferentially accumulates in gray matter synaptasomal and mitochondrial membranes (Suzuki et al., 1997). DHA is mobilized from membrane phospholipids by the calcium-independent phospholipase A2 (iPLA2) isoform (Farooqui and Harrocks, 2004) and free DHA has been found to interact with second messenger signaling pathways associated with synaptic neurotransmission and plasticity (McNamara et al., 2006). It has been estimated that approximately 2-8% of rat brain DHA is replaced daily due to metabolism, and has a loss half-life in total rat brain phospholipids of 33 days under steady state ALA intake (DeMar et al., 2004; Rapoport et al., 2001). Dietary *n*-3 fatty acid insufficiency is associated with reductions in iPLA2 expression and activity, and a >2-fold reduction in the loss half-life of DHA in rat PFC (Demar et al., 2004; Rao et al., 2007a). DHA and its bioactive metabolites have been shown to be neuroprotective against a variety of insults associated with oxidative stress and lipid peroxidation in the fetal (Green et al., 2001; Yavin et al., 2002) and adult (Belayev et al., 2009; Blondeau et al., 2002; Hogyes et al., 2003; Orr et al., 2013; Ozyurt et al., 2007; Wu et al., 2004) rat brain. Increasing dietary LC*n*-3 fatty acid status is also protective against inflammation- (Tuzun et al., 2012) and trauma-induced (Bailes and Mills, 2010) axonal white matter injury in adult rats. This evidence suggests that cortical DHA has protective effects which may be mediated by anti-inflammatory and anti-oxidative mechanisms.

During perinatal rodent brain development, cortical DHA concentrations increase sharply in parallel with active periods of neurogenesis, neuroblast migration, and synaptogenesis (Green and Yavin, 1996). Dietary-induced deficits in brain DHA accrual during perinatal maturation are associated with reductions in neurotrophic factor expression (Ikemoto et al., 2000; Rao et al., 2007b), neurogenesis and migration (Beltz et al., 2007; Kawakita et al., 2006; Yavin et al., 2009), dendritic arborization (Sakamoto et al., 2007), and embryonic cortical plate expansion (Coti Bertrand et al., 2006). Dietary-induced deficits in rat brain DHA accrual during perinatal maturation are also associated with elevated pro-inflammatory signaling molecules in the rat PFC (Rao et al., 2007a), reductions in astrocyte-mediated glucose uptake in the PFC (Pifferi et al., 2005; Ximenes da Silva et al., 2002), and neuronal shrinkage in limbic structures including the hippocampus (Ahmad et al., 2002). Most relevant to cortical circuit maturation, deficits in brain DHA accrual during perinatal development are associated with reductions in neurite outgrowth, synaptogenesis, and synaptic plasticity (Calderon and Kim, 2004; Cao et al., 2009; Ikemoto et al., 1997).

A persistent enhancement of glutamatergic synaptic efficacy exemplified by long-term potentiation (LTP) is thought to mediate the formation of new synaptic connections and requires activation of *N*-methyl-D-aspartate (NMDA) receptors. An early ex vivo study found that DHA enhances the function of glutamate receptor channels (Nishikawa et al., 1994) though the effects of exogenous application of DHA on LTP induction are pathway specific (Fujiti et al., 2001; Itokazu et al., 2000; Mirnikjoo et al., 2001). Nevertheless, *n*-3 fatty acid deprivation during perinatal development is associated with decreases of NMDA receptor NR2A subunit expression, reductions in glutamatergic synapses, and impaired LTP in the rat hippocampus (Cao et al., 2009). It is also relevant that dietary-induced restoration of DHA deficits in the aged rat brain is associated with the normalization of lower NR2B subunit expression and hippocampal LTP deficits (Dyall et al., 2007; Martin et al., 2002; McGahon et al., 1999). Dietary FO fortification attenuates impairment of pre-pulse inhibition following treatment with the NMDA receptor antagonist ketamine (Gama et al., 2012; Zugno et al., 2014) but not histopathological features induced by chronic NMDA treatment (Keleshian et al., 2014). Together, these findings suggest that the accrual and maintenance cortical DHA is required for optimal glutamatergic synaptic neurotransmission, plasticity, and resilience.

Consistent with impaired glutamatergic synaptic plasticity, deficits in brain DHA accrual are associated with impairments in hippocampus-dependent spatial learning which are attenuated with dietary *n*-3 fatty acid fortification (Fedorova et al., 2009; Moriguchi et al., 2000; Moriguchi and Salem, 2003). Perinatal deficits in brain DHA accrual are also associated with learning impairments in olfactory discrimination tasks (Greiner et al., 1999, 2001; Hichami et al., 2007), and the persistence of long-term memories in an inhibitory avoidance task (Bach et al., 2014). In the latter study, memory impairments in *n*-3 fatty acid deficient rats were associated with reductions in NMDA NR2B subunit expression. An ultrastructural study found that *n*-3 fatty acid deprivation led to abnormal decreases in vesicle densities in hippocampal glutamatergic synapses following learning (Yoshida et al., 1997). Naturally occurring reductions in aged rat brain DHA levels are associated with impaired learning performance (Ulmann et al., 2001), and dietary-induced restoration of aged brain DHA content is associated with improvements in hippocampus-dependent learning performance (Carrie et al., 2002). These and other rodent data suggest that cortical DHA accrual and maintenance are required for optimal synaptic plasticity mediating associative learning performance over the lifespan.

Deficits in mesocorticolimbic dopamine synaptic function are thought to contribute to impairments in attention and executive function (Akil et al., 1999; Ernst et al., 1998; Rosa Neto et al., 2002) as well as core symptoms of depression including anhedonia (Nestler and Carlezon, 2006; Stein, 2008). Rat studies have demonstrated that deficits in brain DHA accrual during perinatal development are associated with a significant loss of dopamine neurons in the ventral tegmental area, the source of mesolimbic and mesocortical dopamine projections (Ahmad et al., 2008). Perinatal deficits in brain DHA accrual are also associated with increased expression tyrosine hydroxylase, the rate limiting enzyme in dopamine biosynthesis, in the dorsal striatum of adolescent but not adult rats (Bondi et al., 2014). Perinatal deficits in brain DHA accrual are associated with significant deficits in basal and tyramine-stimulated extracellular dopamine concentrations in the frontal cortex of young adult rats (Kodas et al., 2002a; Zimmer et al., 1998). Importantly, deficits in tyramine-stimulated dopamine release are reversible with early (P0-P14), but not later (P21), postnatal *n*-3 fatty acid supplementation (Kodas et al., 2002a). Rats subjected to perinatal deficits in brain DHA accrual also exhibit deficits in mesolimbic dopamine neurotransmission (Zimmer et al., 2000b, 2002). Perinatal deficits in brain DHA accrual also leads to alterations in dopamine D1 and D2 receptor expression and binding (Delion et al., 1996; Kuperstein et al., 2008; Zimmer et al., 2000b) but does not significantly alter the density or function of dopamine transporters (Kodas et al., 2002b). Our group has additionally found that dietary-induced deficits in PFC DHA accrual during peri-adolescent development is sufficient to significantly reduce dopamine D2 receptor binding density, but not binding affinity or mRNA expression, in the young adult PFC (Figure 3). Maternal dietary FO supplementation throughout gestation and lactation significantly increases dopamine concentrations in the frontal cortex of adult offspring (Chalon et al., 1998). These findings suggest that early perinatal brain DHA accrual is critical for the functional maturation of mesocortical and mesolimbic dopamine pathways.

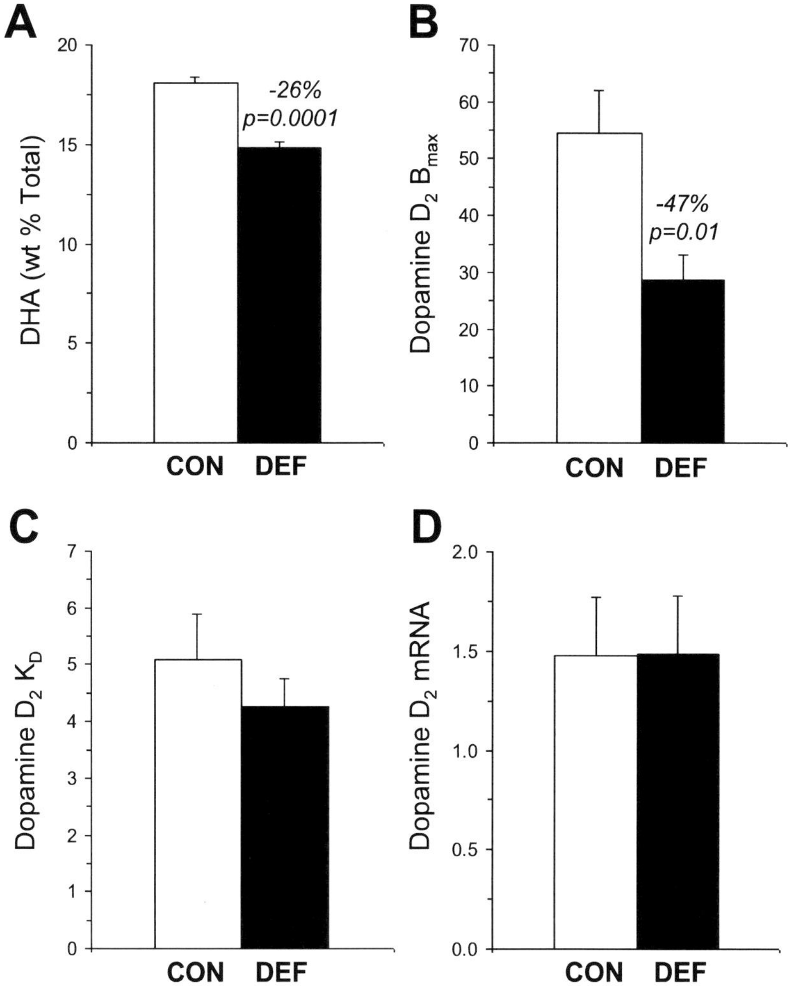

Figure 3. Effects of dietary *n*-3 fatty acid (ALA) depletion initiated prior to adolescence (postnatal day 21-90) on DHA levels (A), dopamine D2 receptor binding density (Bmax)(B), dopamine D2 receptor binding affinity (KD)(C), and dopamine D2 receptor mRNA expression (D) in the young adult PFC. Note that dietary *n*-3 fatty acid insufficiency and associated PFC DHA deficits are associated with lower dopamine D2 receptor binding density in the young adulthood rat PFC. Values are group means ± S.E.M.

Pharmacological studies have additionally found that deficits in perinatal brain DHA accrual are associated with altered responses to drugs that target dopamine neurotransmission and commonly used to treat ADHD (amphetamine) and psychosis (haloperidol). For example, amphetamine-induced locomotor activity was significantly enhanced in *n*-3 fatty acid deficient rats (Levant et al., 2004), and amphetamine-induced behavioral sensitization is significantly augmented in *n*-3 fatty acid deficient adult C57BL/6J mice (McNamara et al., 2008c). Moreover, amphetamine-induced behavioral sensitization was significantly augmented by n-3 fatty acid deficiency in a 'sensitization-resistant' inbred mouse strain (McNamara et al., 2008d). In the latter study, augmented sensitization was associated with greater amphetamine-induced mesolimbic dopamine activity. Our group has additionally found that dietary-induced deficits in rat PFC DHA accrual initiated prior to the adolescent period is sufficient to significantly augment amphetamine-induced behavioral sensitization in young adult rats, and additionally found that this augmented response is associated with reduced dopamine turnover in the PFC (Figure 4). Sensorimotor gating as measured by pre-pulse inhibition of the acoustic startle response is impaired by amphetamine (Mansbach et al., 1988) and perinatal deficits in brain DHA accrual (Fedorova et al., 2009). Perinatal deficits in cortical DHA accrual are associated significant decrements in catalepsy induced by the dopamine D2 receptor antagonist haloperidol (Levant et al., 2004). Therefore, pharmacological studies provide further evidence that n-3 fatty acid deficiency leads to robust abnormalities in dopamine synaptic transmission.

Consistent with clinical evidence implicating a dysregulation in serotonin (5-hydroxytryptamine, 5-HT) synaptic transmission in the pathophysiology and treatment of depression and aggression (Arango et al., 2002; Coccaro et al., 1997; Vaswani et al., 2003), post-weaning deficits in cortical DHA accrual are associated with elevated behavioral indices of aggression and depression in rats (DeMar et al., 2006). Interestingly, dietary FO fortification significantly decreases depression-like behavior similar to selective serotonin reuptake inhibitor (SSRI) medications in the forced swimming test (Carlezon et al., 2005; Huang et al., 2008). Moreover, the combination of dietary FO supplementation and fluoxetine is significantly more effective than fluoxetine treatment alone for reducing depression-like behavior in the forced swim test (Laino et al., 2010; Lakhwani et al., 2007). Although post-weaning deficits in cortical DHA accrual are not associated with diminished SSRI efficacy in female rats in the forced swim test (McNamara et al., 2013a), it is associated with abnormal behavioral activation in the forced swim test in male rats (Able et al., 2014). These findings suggest that cortical DHA status is an important determinant of behaviors regulated by serotonin including depression and aggression.

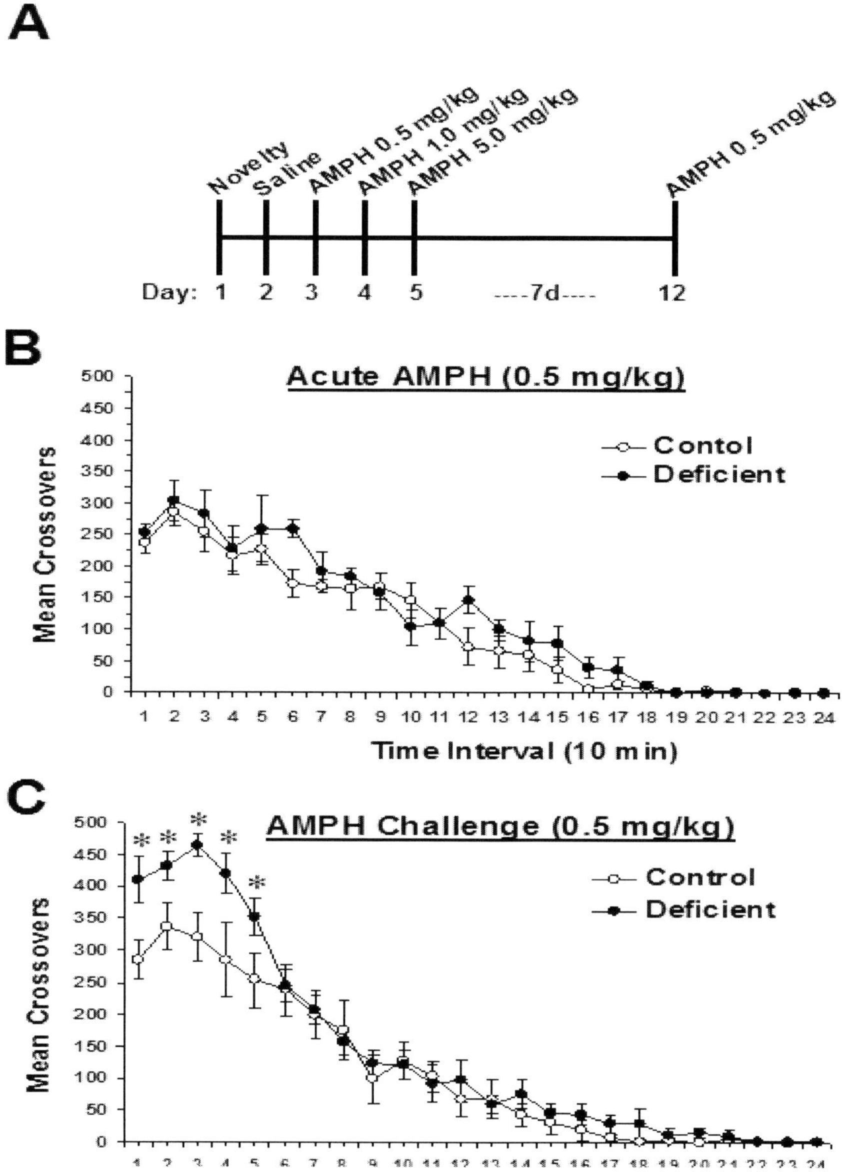

Figure 4. (Continued.)

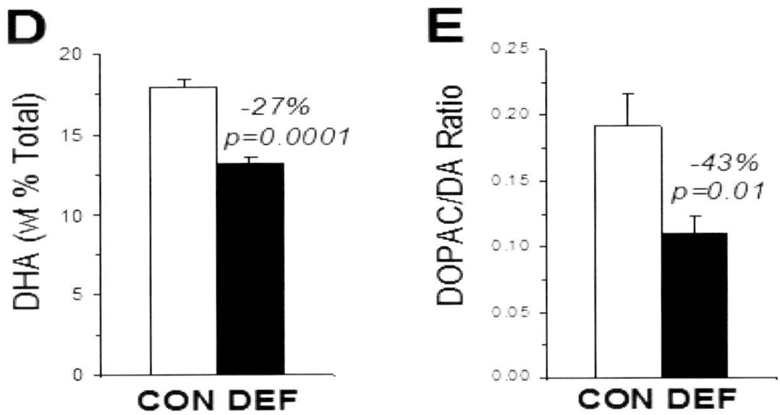

Figure 4. Effects of dietary *n*-3 fatty acid insufficiency during adolescence (post-natal day 21-90) on ampheta-mine (AMPH)-induced beha-vioral (locomotor activity) sensitization and dopamine metabolism in the young adulthood rat PFC. The escalating AMPH dose schedule is presented in (A). In response to acute low-dose AMPH (0.5 mg/kg), rats fed the control diet (*n*-3 fatty acid fortified, n=8) and *n*-3 fatty acid deficient diet (n=8) exhibit similar elevations in locomotor activity (B). Following treatment with escalating AMPH doses, low-dose AMPH (0.5 mg/kg) induces significantly greater locomotor activity in rats fed the *n*-3 fatty acid depleted diet compared with controls (C). PFC DHA levels are presented in (D) and PFC dopamine metabolism (dihydroxy-phenylacetic acid (DOPAC)/ dopamine (DA) ratio) determined immediately following the AMPH challenge is presented in (E). Values are group means ± S.E.M. *$p \leq 0.05$ vs. Controls.

Maternal dietary FO fortification significantly increases serotonin concentrations in the frontal cortex (Chalon et al., 1998) and attenuates reductions in frontal cortex serotonin content in response to chronic stress (Vancassel et al., 2008) in young adult offspring. Conversely, perinatal deficits in cortical DHA accrual are associated with impaired fenfluramine-induced elevations in extracellular serotonin concentrations (Kodas et al., 2004), reductions in midbrain expression of tryptophan hydroxylase-2, the rate-limiting enzyme in serotonin biosynthesis (McNamara et al., 2009a), and elevations in 5-HT2A receptor binding density in the rat frontal cortex (Delion et al., 1996). The 5-HIAA/5-HT ratio, an index of serotonin turnover, was significantly increased in the frontal cortex, hypothalamus, and ventral striatum of adult perinatal *n*-3-deficient rats and was prevented by early normalization of *n*-3 fatty acid status (McNamara et al., 2010c). Importantly, the increase in the 5-HIAA/5-HT ratio observed in the perinatal DHA-deficient rat brain is opposite to that produced by the selective serotonin reuptake inhibitor (SSRI) antidepressant medication fluoxetine (McNamara et al., 2013a). Together this evidence suggests that LC*n*-3 fatty acid status during development is an important determinant of central serotonin synaptic transmission in adult rats.

4. Non-Human Primate Neurodevelopment

In the developing monkey brain, frontal cortex DHA concentrations represent ~15% of total fatty acids at birth, and between birth and 22 months of age increase to comprise ~22% of total fatty acids (Anderson et al., 2005; Neuringer et al., 1986). Feeding studies have found that a maternal diet low in ALA beginning 2 months prior to conception is associated with reduced neonatal monkey prefrontal cortex DHA concentrations at birth compared with neonates whose mothers were maintained on a standard diet containing higher levels of ALA (Anderson et al., 2005; Neuringer et al., 1986). Postnatal dietary FO or ALA fortification leads to a progressive normalization of prefrontal cortex DHA concentrations in DHA-deficient neonatal monkeys (Anderson et al., 2005; Connor et al., 1990). Baboons born preterm exhibit cortical DHA deficits compared with term births, and 4 week feeding with DHA-fortified human infant formula is more efficient for normalizing cortical DHA levels than is human infant formula not fortified with DHA (Sarkadi-Nagy et al., 2003, 2004). These studies suggest that gestational length and maternal DHA status, as well as postnatal dietary DHA intake, are critical determinants of cortical DHA status of young adult non-human primates.

Primate perinatal *n*-3 fatty acid deficiency is associated with deficits in visual attention (Reisbick et al., 1997), polydipsia (excessive thirst) (Reisbick et al., 1990), and deficits in visual acuity and electroretinogram abnormalities (Anderson et al., 2005; Neuringer et al., 1986). Electroretinogram abnormalities have also been observed in neonatal baboons born preterm (Diau et al., 2003). Consistent with elevated mesolimbic dopamine activity, perinatal *n*-3 fatty acid deficiency is associated increased home cage stereotypy and locomotion bouts (Reisbick et al., 1994). A positron emission tomography (PET) study demonstrated that dietary supplementation with DHA improves the age-related impairment in cerebral blood flow in somatosensory cortex in response to tactile stimulation (Tsukada et al., 2000). Importantly, a recent neuroimaging study found that resting-state functional connectivity among prefrontal cortical networks was deficient in monkeys raised on an *n*-3 fatty acid deficient diet compared with monkeys raised on FO fortified diet (Grayson et al., 2014). These findings provide functional evidence that lower cortical DHA status is associated with deficits in cortical circuit maturation and a range of neurodevelopmental abnormalities in young adult non-human primates.

5. HUMAN NEURODEVELOPMENT

During pregnancy the developing human fetus acquires DHA from maternal stores, and DHA is preferentially transported across the human placenta by fatty acid transport proteins (Dutta-Roy, 2000; Koletzko et al., 2007). Emerging clinical evidence suggests that ovarian hormones positively regulate ALA→DHA conversion (Bakewell et al., 2006; Burdge and Wooton, 2002) and that ALA→DHA biosynthesis is more efficient in pregnant women and infants compared with healthy adult human subjects (Brenna et al., 2009; Otto et al., 2001). During human neonatal development, DHA accumulates in brain tissue at a rapid rate during the third trimester in association with active periods of neurogenesis, neuroblast migration, differentiation and synaptogenesis (Clandinin et al., 1980a; Martinez, 1992). Some observational studies suggest that higher maternal DHA status or higher seafood intake during pregnancy has a beneficial effect on term infant neurodevelopmental outcomes, including more mature sleep patterns, higher visual acuity, faster processing speed, lower distractibility, higher stereoacuity and visual attention (Helland et al., 2003; Cheruku et al., 2002; Williams et al., 2001; Colombo et al., 2004; Innis et al., 2001b). However, recent controlled trials have found that maternal DHA supplementation during pregnancy do not have a significant impact on visual acuity (Smithers et al., 2011) or neurocognitive outcomes (Makrides et al., 2010) in term infants at 18 months of age.

Higher maternal DHA and fetal status during pregnancy is an important determinant of gestational length and intrauterine growth (Carlson et al., 2013; Olsen et al., 1992, 2007; Salvig and Lamont, 2011). As observed in non-human primates (Sarkadi-Nagy et al., 2003), human infants born preterm exhibit lower erythrocyte and postmortem cortical DHA concentrations compared with term infants fed the same ALA-fortified formula postpartum (Clandinin et al., 1980a; Farquharson et al., 1992, 1995; Martinez, 1992; Martinez and Mougan, 1998). Preterm infants fed formulas without DHA also have lower erythrocyte and postmortem cerebral cortex DHA levels compared with preterm infants fed human milk (Carlson et al., 1986; Farquharson et al., 1992, 1995; Martinez, 1992). Children and adolescents born preterm also exhibit a significantly higher incidence of attention deficits, impulsivity, learning disability, language impairments, hyperactivity, anxiety, motor impairments, and poor social functioning relative to age- and sex-matched term children/adolescents (Bhutta et al., 2002; Foulder-Hughes and Cooke, 2003). Importantly, preterm birth is associated with increased risk for developing ADHD in childhood (Bhutta et al., 2002; Botting et al., 1997; Johnson et al., 2010) and mood and psychotic disorders during adolescence and young adulthood (Nosarti et al., 2012).

Postpartum the human fetal brain continues to grow from ~350 g at birth to ~925 g at 1 year of age (Dobbing and Sands, 1973), during which DHA represents approximately 9% of total cortical fatty acid composition (Carver et al., 2001; Clandinin et al., 1980b). Postpartum neonates are reliant on maternal breast milk (or formula) as the sole source of DHA. Human breast milk DHA concentrations are highly correlated with maternal dietary DHA but not ALA intake (Francois et al., 2003; Lauritzen et al., 2002; Jensen et al., 2000), and vary widely across different countries in accordance with habitual dietary fish consumption (Brenna et al., 2007). Term infants fed formulas without DHA consistently exhibit significantly lower erythrocyte or postmortem brain cortex DHA concentrations relative to breastfed infants or infants fed formula containing DHA (Putnam et al., 1982; Auestad et al., 1997; Byard et al., 1995; Farquharson et al., 1995; Gibson et al., 1996; Jamieson et al., 1999; Makrides et al., 1994). The effect of postnatal DHA supplementation on neurocognitive development in term infants has been reviewed in detail previously (Carlson, 2009; Scholtz et al., 2013). Although controversial, studies have found that infants fed formulas without DHA exhibit several neurological and neurocognitive 'soft signs' in infancy and childhood compared with infants fed formulas with DHA or maternal breast milk, including lower visual acuity, slower processing speed on tests of visual recognition memory, more mature motor movement, problem-solving, and psychomotor function.

During early childhood development DHA levels continue to increase in the frontal cortex (Carver et al., 2001) in association with linear increases in frontal cortex gray matter expansion (Giedd et al., 2009; Paus et al., 1999; Sowell et al., 1999) and the maturation of frontal-mediated neurocognitive processes including attention and executive function (Conklin et al., 2007). A recent observational study found that greater LC*n*-3 fatty acid intake measured by questionnaire was associated with better hippocampus-dependent relational memory performance in 52 children aged 7-9 years of age (Baym et al., 2014).

However, the results of acute LCn-3 fatty acid supplementation trials have in general not observed significant neurocognitive benefits in healthy developing children (Ryan et al., 2010). For example, a controlled trial of 450 healthy children 8-10 years of age found that 16-week treatment with 400 mg FO did not significantly impact performance across several cognitive tasks (Kirby et al., 2010). A more recent controlled trial of 362 healthy children 7-9 years of age found that 16-week treatment with 600 mg DHA did not influence teacher-rated behavior or working memory performance, but was associated with improved reading performance in a subgroup of 224 children with poor reading ability (Richardson et al., 2012). In the latter study, DHA supplementation was associated with reduced parent-rated ADHD-type symptoms including oppositional behavior and hyperactivity. The results from these and other short-term LCn-3 fatty acid supplementation trials suggest no robust neurocognitive benefits in healthy developing children, though additional longer dose-ranging studies in children with initially low DHA status are warranted.

Prospective longitudinal studies have begun to investigate the relationship between maternal LCn-3 fatty acid intake and neurodevelopmental outcomes in older children. One study found that supplementing pregnant and lactating women with FO resulted in higher IQ scores at 4 years of age compared with maternal supplementation with corn oil (Helland et al., 2003). However, a follow-up study found that maternal FO supplementation during pregnancy and lactation did not impact IQ at 7 years of age (Helland et al., 2008). Another study found that maternal FO supplementation during the first 4 months of lactation did not result in statistically significant effects at 7 years of age on neurocognitive outcomes including working memory and inhibitory control compared with olive oil supplementation (Cheatham et al., 2011). Moreover, a large trial found that maternal DHA supplementation during pregnancy did not significantly impact cognition, language, and executive function at 4 years of age (Makrides et al., 2014). However, the Avon Longitudinal Study of Parents and Children (ALSPAC) found that higher fish consumption during pregnancy was associated with higher scores of fine motor skills, verbal IQ, social development, and pro-social behavior in children 7-8 years of age (Hibbeln et al., 2007). While these data suggest that higher fetal DHA status may have long-term beneficial effects on neurocognitive outcomes in childhood, variability in dietary DHA intake during the intervening period may contribute to variability between studies.

Prospective longitudinal studies have also investigated the relationship between fetal cord blood DHA levels and neurodevelopmental outcomes in older children. Studies have found that higher cord blood DHA levels are associated with higher movement scores but not neurocognitive scores at 7 years of age (Bakker et al., 2003; 2009), better visual function at 5 years of age (Jacques et al., 2011), and better recognition memory and associated event-related potentials at ~11 years of age (Boucher et al., 2011). Another study found that higher cord blood DHA or LC*n*-3 fatty acid levels were associated with lower parent-reported hyperactivity/inattention and emotional symptoms among 416 children at 10 years of age (Kohlboeck et al., 2011). Lastly, a longitudinal study found that higher cord blood DHA status was associated with lower levels of internalizing emotional problems including depression and externalizing conduct problems among 393 children at 7 years of age in subjects fed DHA-free formula but not those fed human milk (Krabbendam et al., 2007). The latter finding suggests that increasing postnatal dietary DHA intake can mitigate the emergence of psychiatric problems in youth exposed to low DHA levels *in utero*.

During adolescent development cortical DHA levels continue to increase to ~15% total cortical fatty acids in young adulthood (Carver et al., 2001) and this increase coincides with frontal cortex synaptic pruning (Glantz et al., 2007; Huttenlocher, 1979; Petanjek et al., 2011), and white matter expansion and frontal lobe functional connectivity (Ducharme et al., 2012; Giedd et al., 2009; Paus et al., 1999; Sowell et al., 1999; Tisserand et al., 2002). Adolescence is a period of increasing dietary autonomy and surveys have found that a large percentage of adolescents residing in western countries consume low quantities of LC*n*-3 fatty acids in their habitual diet (Clayton et al., 2009a; Harel et al., 2001; Lauritzen et al., 2012; Sichert-Hellert et al., 2009). For example, a survey of 1,117 ninth-grade adolescents (average age 15 years) in the United States found that only 36 percent consumed fish at least once a week, 29 percent consumed fish once a month, and 35 percent consumed fish <3 times per year (Harel et al., 2001). Importantly, lower LC*n*-3 fatty acid intake by adolescents is associated with a higher prevalence of depressive symptoms (Allen et al., 2013; Murakami et al., 2010; Oddy et al., 2011; Swenne et al., 2011) and potentially psychosis in ultra-high risk youth (Amminger et al., 2010). Although there is currently little known about the importance of LC*n*-3 fatty acid intake during childhood on cognitive outcomes in adolescence, a longitudinal cohort study found that greater fish intake (>1 time per week) at 15 years of age was associated with higher scores in composite IQ and verbal performance and visuospatial performance at 18 years of age compared with adolescents consuming fish >1 time per week (Aberg et al., 2009).

6. Neuroimaging

Human neuroimaging studies indicate that the childhood and adolescent period is associated with the maturation of frontal cortical regions that mediate attention and executive function and the establishment of structural and functional connectivity between frontal regions and limbic structures that mediate emotion and mood (Giedd et al., 2009; Paus et al., 1999; Sowell et al., 1999). Reciprocal connections between the PFC and limbic structures including the amygdala are mediated in part by the uncinate fasciculus and superior longitudinal fasciculus (Figure 5A) which negatively gate amygdala outputs to the hypothalamus and nucleus accumbens (Ebeling and Von Cramon, 1992; Kier et al., 2004). A recent neuroimaging study found that resting-state functional connectivity among prefrontal cortical networks was deficient in monkeys raised on an *n*-3 fatty acid deficient diet compared with monkeys raised on FO fortified diet (Grayson et al., 2014). Moreover, structural imaging studies have also found that children and adolescents born preterm, which is associated with deficits in fetal cortical DHA accrual, exhibit significant reductions in regional cortical gray matter volumes, reduced amygdala and hippocampal volumes, reduced corpus callosum and white matter volumes, and larger cerebral ventricles (Kesler et al., 2008; Nagy et al., 2003; Nosarti et al., 2002; Ment et al., 2009; Peterson et al., 2000; Stewart et al., 1999). More recent imaging studies have also found that children, adolescents, and adults born preterm exhibit decreased white matter tract integrity and reduced connectivity within cortical networks (Constable et al., 2008; Gozzo et al., 2009; Lubsen et al., 2011; Mullen et al., 2011; Schafer et al., 2009; Smyser et al., 2013; White et al., 2014). Together, these translational imaging findings suggest that reduced cortical DHA accrual during perinatal development increase risk for enduring deficits in cortical circuit maturation.

As discussed above, patients with psychiatric disorders including ADHD and mood or psychotic disorders exhibit peripheral and potentially central DHA deficits compared with healthy subjects. Similar to children and adolescents born preterm, patients with ADHD exhibit decreased white matter tract integrity (Chuang et al., 2013; Lawrence et al., 2013; Silk et al., 2009) and reduced connectivity within frontal lobe cortical networks (Cao et al., 2009; Sun et al., 2012; Tian et al., 2006). Patients with mood (Adler et al., 2006; Bellani and Brambilla, 2011; Bora et al., 2012; Cullen et al., 2010; Dickstein et al., 2010; Guo et al., 2012; Lin et al., 2011b; Sacher et al., 2012; Strakowski et al., 2012) or psychotic (Canu et al., 2014; De Peri et al., 2012; Vita et al., 2013; Colombo et al., 2012) disorders also exhibit decreased frontal white matter tract integrity and reduced connectivity within cortical networks. These findings suggest that major psychiatric disorders that are associated with blood DHA deficits and initially emerge during childhood and adolescence are associated with aberrant brain organization characterized by suboptimal cortical circuit development.

Additional evidence from human MRI studies further suggests a beneficial effect of LC*n*-3 fatty acids on cortical structure and function over the lifespan (McNamara, 2013b). For example, in a controlled functional MRI trial our group investigated the effects of 8-week DHA supplementation on cortical activity during performance of sustained attention task (CPT-IP) in healthy male children (McNamara et al., 2010d). At 8 weeks, erythrocyte membrane DHA composition increased significantly from baseline in subjects receiving DHA but not placebo (Figure 5B). During sustained attention, subjects receiving DHA exhibited significantly greater change from baseline in the activation of dorsolateral PFC (BA9), and greater decreases in the cerebellar cortex, relative to placebo. Using a less stringent statistical threshold, greater increases in the PFC (Figure 5C) and greater decreases in temporal cortex (Figure 5D) were observed in the DHA group compared with placebo. These preliminary fMRI findings suggest that increasing DHA status during development may augment functional connectivity within frontolimbic networks.

Proton magnetic resonance spectroscopy (^{1}H MRS) is a voxel-based technique that determines in vivo cortical concentrations of different compounds associated with cortical integrity and metabolism. For example, *myo*-inositol (mI) is metabolized from glucose via 1L-myo-inositol 1-phosphate synthase and is predominantly concentrated in astroctyes, and *N*-acetyl aspartate (NAA) is primarily localized to neurons and is positively correlated with mitochondrial metabolism (Brand et al., 1993; Griffin et al., 2002). ^{1}H MRS studies have consistently observed lower NAA concentrations in human cortical infarcts during the acute or subacute phase of ischemia (Lanfermann et al., 1995).

In a preclinical ^{1}H MRS study, our group found that perinatal deficits in brain DHA accrual were associated with reductions in mI, but not NAA, in the rat PFC (McNamara et al., 2009b). In a clinical ^{1}H MRS study employing healthy developing male children, we recently reported that subjects with low erythrocyte DHA status exhibited lower mI and NAA concentrations in the anterior cingulate cortex compared with subjects in the high erythrocyte DHA status group (McNamara et al., 2013). A preliminary placebo-controlled ^{1}H MRS study found that 12-week supplementation with EPA selectively increased NAA concentrations in the anterior cingulate cortex of medicated patients with bipolar disorder (Frangou et al., 2007). These preliminary ^{1}H MRS data are consistent with DHA status being positively associated with cortical neuronal (NAA) and astrocyte (mI) integrity.

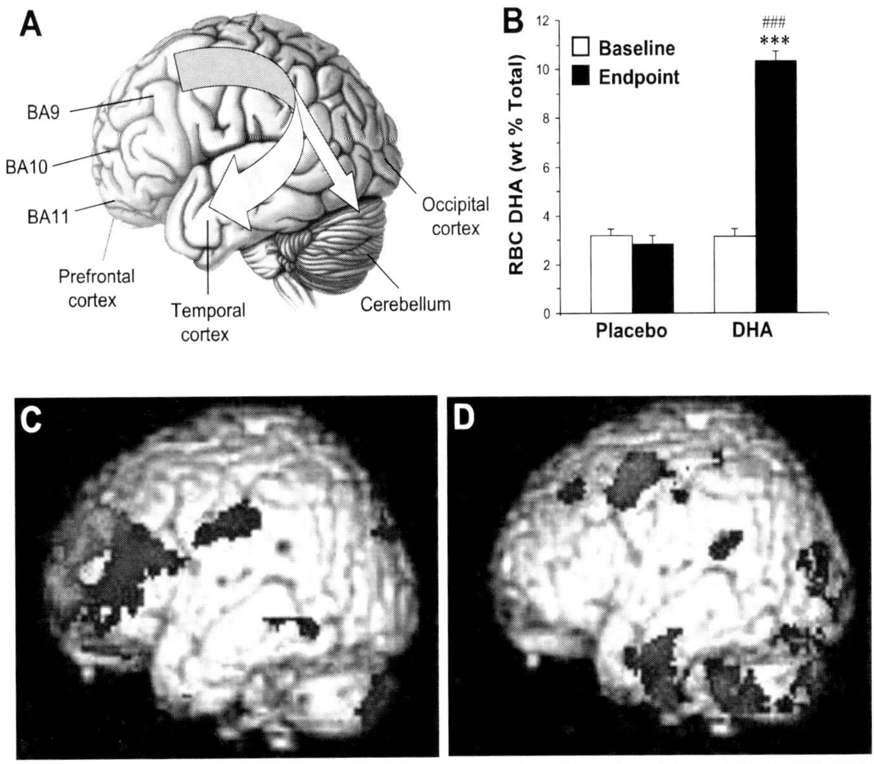

Figure 5. (A) Diagram illustrating the human PFC and major subdivisions (BA9 - DLPFC, BA10 - orbitofrontal cortex, BA11 - ventrolateral PFC) and the white matter bundles (i.e., superior longitudinal fasciculus) linking the PFC with temporal lobe structures and the cerebellum (arrows). (B) Erythrocyte membrane DHA composition of healthy male children (aged 8-10 years) treated with placebo (n=10) or DHA (1200 mg/d, n=13) at baseline and study endpoint (8 weeks). Functional t-maps illustrating group (placebo vs. DHA) differences in baseline-to-endpoint change in regional activation (positive BOLD, DHA > placebo) (C) and deactivation (negative BOLD, placebo > DHA)(D) during performance of a sustained attention task (CPT-IP). The color gradient (red → yellow) reflects increasing statistical significance relative to placebo ($P \leq 0.05$ threshold and $T \leq 25$ cluster volume). Note that subjects receiving DHA exhibit greater baseline-to-endpoint increases in PFC activity and greater baseline-to-endpoint decreases in temporal cortex and cerebellum activity compared with subjects receiving placebo. In (B) values are group mean ± S.E.M. ***$P \leq 0.001$ vs. baseline, ###$P \leq 0.001$ vs. placebo at endpoint.

Emerging evidence from structural neuroimaging studies further support a beneficial effect of LC*n*-3 fatty acids on cortical integrity over the lifespan (Conklin et al., 2007; Samieri et al., 2012; Titova et al., 2013; Virtanen et al., 2013; Walhovd et al., 2013). For example, one study found that greater habitual dietary LC*n*-3 fatty acid intake, which is positively correlated with erythrocyte DHA composition, was associated with larger cortical gray matter volumes in several corticolimbic regions including the anterior cingulate cortex, hippocampus, and amygdala (Conklin et al., 2007). It is relevant, therefore, that patients with psychiatric disorders commonly exhibit gray matter volume deficits in the anterior cingulate cortex, hippocampus, and amygdala (Castellanos et al., 2002; Glahn et al., 2008; Kempton et al., 2011). While this preliminary imaging evidence suggests that LC*n*-3 fatty acid status is positively correlated with cortical structural integrity, additional research is needed to determine whether deficits cortical integrity observed in patients with psychiatric disorders can be reversed or prevented by increasing LC*n*-3 fatty acid status.

CONCLUSION

Over the past 30 years a body of evidence has emerged from animal and clinical studies which support the general assertion that normal brain development requires optimal DHA levels. Rodent studies suggest that cortical DHA has neurotrophic and neuroprotective properties, and that reductions in perinatal rat brain DHA accrual are associated with delays in neuronal migration and arborization, synaptic pathology, and deficits in multiple neurotransmitter systems including glutamate, dopamine, and serotonin. Deficits in perinatal rat brain DHA accrual also lead to neurocognitive impairments and elevated behavioral indices of depression and aggression. Non-human primate studies further suggest a link between *n*-3 fatty acid deficiency during perinatal development and long-standing deficits in functional connectivity within cortical networks, hyperactivity, and impairments in visual attention. In general, results from animal studies provide strong evidence for a critical role of perinatal DHA accrual for the normal maturation of neural circuits mediating cognitive and emotional processes.

Human studies suggest that preterm birth, which results in deficits in third trimester fetal cortical DHA accrual, is associated with enduring abnormalities in brain structure and function including connectivity deficits within cortical networks, and a spectrum of neurocognitive impairments particularly in attention and executive function. Preterm birth is also associated with increased risk for psychiatric disorders including ADHD, psychosis, and mood disorders which are also associated with deficits in functional connectivity within cortical networks. Moreover, early postnatal DHA supplementation has been found in some studies to improve visual acuity and visual attention processes in infants and children born preterm. These associations suggest that third trimester cortical DHA accrual may play a critical role in the maturation of cortical networks mediating cognitive and emotional processes. While prospective longitudinal studies are needed to evaluate whether early LC*n*-3 fatty acid supplementation can reduce the risk of developing psychiatric disorders in children and adolescence born preterm, some prospective longitudinal studies have observed a positive relationship between fetal cord blood DHA levels and neurodevelopmental and psychiatric outcomes in older children.

While it is not currently known whether LC*n*-3 fatty acid supplementation alone is sufficient to modify functional connectivity within cortical networks once established, it appears to play a critical role in their initial development. This is directly supported by a recent non-human primate study finding that *n*-3 fatty acid deficiency during perinatal development is associated with long-standing hypoactivity in functional connectivity within prefrontal cortical circuits. Moreover, emerging neuroimaging evidence indicates that psychiatric disorders that initially emerge in childhood and adolescence are also associated with frontal structural and functional connectivity deficits and low blood DHA levels compared with healthy developing youth. These translational findings suggest a potential link between low LC*n*-3 fatty acid status and deficits in the development of functional connectivity within prefrontal cortical networks. Although LC*n*-3 fatty acid supplementation has been found to improve symptoms in patients with psychiatric disorders, it is not known whether this effect in mediated by increasing functional connectivity within cortical circuits. It remains possible that cortical circuit maturation deficits secondary to LC*n*-3 fatty acid deficits may represent a permanent neurodevelopmental 'scar' that is potentially irreversible once established. Additional neuroimaging studies are warranted to determine whether early long-term LC*n*-3 fatty acid supplementation can restore normal functional connectivity with cortical networks in youth with or at high risk for developing psychiatric disorders.

The role of perinatal brain DHA accrual on the maturation of cortical circuitry is only beginning to be fully understood. Extant evidence from translational studies suggest that optimal brain development and function requires an optimal level of LC*n*-3 fatty acids during perinatal development, and maternal and offspring LC*n*-3 fatty acid deficiency is associated with increased risk of preterm birth, deficits in functional connectivity with cortical circuits, and ensuing cognitive impairments and emotional dysregulation. Developing a more comprehensive understanding of the requirement for LC*n*-3 fatty acids during normal human perinatal brain development could therefore have significant implications for informing optimal intake levels during critical periods of neurodevelopment, and may represent a novel preventative strategy for youth who were born preterm and are at increased risk for developing psychiatric disorders.

Acknowledgments

This work was supported in part by National Institute of Health grants AG034617 and DK097599 to R.K.M. R.K.M. has received research support from NARSAD, Martek Biosciences Inc, The Inflammation Research Foundation (IRF), Ortho-McNeil Janssen, AstraZeneca, Eli Lilly, and was a member of the IRF scientific advisory board.

References

Aberg MA, Aberg N, Brisman J, Sundberg R, Winkvist A, and Torén K. Fish intake of Swedish male adolescents is a predictor of cognitive performance. *Acta Paediatr.* 2009;98:555-560.

Able JA, Liu Y, Jandacek R, Rider T, Tso P, and McNamara RK. Omega-3 fatty acid deficient male rats exhibit abnormal behavioral activation in the forced swim test following chronic fluoxetine treatment: association with altered 5-HT1A and alpha2A adrenergic receptor expression. *J Psychiatr Res.* 2014;50:42-50.

Adler CM, Adams J, DelBello MP, Holland SK, Schmithorst V, Levine A, Jarvis K, and Strakowski SM. Evidence of white matter pathology in bipolar disorder adolescents experiencing their first episode of mania: a diffusion tensor imaging study. *Am J Psychiatry.* 2006;163:322-324.

Ahmad A, Moriguchi T, and Salem N. Decrease in neuron size in docosahexaenoic acid-deficient brain. *Pediatr Neurol.* 2002;26:210-218.

Ahmad SO, Park JH, Radel JD, and Levant B. Reduced numbers of dopamine neurons in the substantia nigra pars compacta and ventral tegmental area of rats fed an *n*-3 polyunsaturated fatty acid-deficient diet: a stereological study. *Neurosci Lett.* 2008;438:303-307.

Akil M, Pierri JN, Whitehead RE, Edgar CL, Mohila C, Sampson AR, and Lewis DA. Lamina-specific alterations in the dopamine innervation of the prefrontal cortex in schizophrenic subjects. *Am J Psychiatry.* 1999;156:1580-1589.

Allen KL, Mori TA, Beilin L, Byrne SM, Hickling S, and Oddy WH. Dietary intake in population-based adolescents: support for a relationship between eating disorder symptoms, low fatty acid intake and depressive symptoms. *J Hum Nutr Diet.* 2013;26:459-469.

Amminger GP, Schäfer MR, Papageorgiou K, Klier CM, Cotton SM, Harrigan SM, Mackinnon A, McGorry PD, and Berger GE. Long-chain omega-3 fatty acids for indicated prevention of psychotic disorders: a randomized, placebo-controlled trial. *Arch Gen Psychiatry.* 2010;67:146-154.

Anderson GJ, Neuringer M, Lin DS, and Connor WE. Can prenatal *N*-3 fatty acid deficiency be completely reversed after birth? Effects on retinal and brain biochemistry and visual function in rhesus monkeys. *Pediatr Res.* 2005;58:865-872.

Angst F, Stassen HH, Clayton PJ, and Angst J. Mortality of patients with mood disorders: follow-up over 34-38 years. *J Affect Disord.* 2002;68:167-181.

Arango V, Underwood MD, and Mann JJ. Serotonin brain circuits involved in major depression and suicide. *Prog Brain Res.* 2002;136:443-453.

Astorg P, Couthouis A, Bertrais S, Arnault N, Meneton P, Guesnet P, Alessandri JM, Galan P, and Hercberg S. Association of fish and long-chain *n*-3 polyunsaturated fatty acid intakes with the occurrence of depressive episodes in middle-aged French men and women. *Prostaglandins Leukot Essent Fatty Acids.* 2008;78:171-182.

Auestad N, Montalto MB, Hall RT, Fitzgerald KM, Wheeler RE, Connor WE, Neuringer M, Connor SL, Taylor JA, and Hartmann EE. Visual acuity, erythrocyte fatty acid composition, and growth in term infants fed formulas with long chain polyunsaturated fatty acids for one year. Ross Pediatric Lipid Study. Pediatr Res. 1997;41:1-10.

Ayuso-Gutierrez JL and del Rio Vega JM. Factors influencing relapse in the long-term course of schizophrenia. *Schizophr Res.* 1997;28:199-206.

Bach SA, de Siqueira LV, Müller AP, Oses JP, Quatrim A, Emanuelli T, Vinadé L, Souza DO, and Moreira JD. Dietary omega-3 deficiency reduces BDNF content and activation NMDA receptor and Fyn in dorsal hippocampus: Implications on persistence of long-term memory in rats. *Nutr Neurosci.* 2014;17:186-192.

Bailes JE and Mills JD. Docosahexaenoic acid reduces traumatic axonal injury in a rodent head injury model. *J Neurotrauma.* 2010;27:1617-1624.

Bakewell L, Burdge GC, and Calder PC. Polyunsaturated fatty acid concentrations in young men and women consuming their habitual diets. *Br J Nutr.* 2006;96:93-99.

Bakker EC, Ghys AJ, Kester AD, Vles JS, Dubas JS, Blanco CE, and Hornstra G. Long-chain polyunsaturated fatty acids at birth and cognitive function at 7 y of age. *Eur J Clin Nutr.* 2003;57:89-95.

Bakker EC, Hornstra G, Blanco CE, and Vles JS. Relationship between long-chain polyunsaturated fatty acids at birth and motor function at 7 years of age. *Eur J Clin Nutr.* 2009;63:499-504.

Barceló-Coblijn G, Murphy EJ, Othman R, Moghadasian MH, Kashour T, and Friel JK. Flaxseed oil and fish-oil capsule consumption alters human red blood cell *n*-3 fatty acid composition: a multiple-dosing trial comparing 2 sources of *n*-3 fatty acid. *Am J Clin Nutr.* 2008;88:801-809.

Baym CL, Khan NA, Monti JM, Raine LB, Drollette ES, Moore RD, Scudder MR, Kramer AF, Hillman CH, and Cohen NJ. Dietary lipids are differentially associated with hippocampal-dependent relational memory in prepubescent children. *Am J Clin Nutr.* 2014;99:1026-1032.

Belayev L, Khoutorova L, Atkins KD, and Bazan NG. Robust docosahexaenoic acid-mediated neuroprotection in a rat model of transient, focal cerebral ischemia. *Stroke.* 2009;40:3121-3126.

Bellani M and Brambilla P. Diffusion imaging studies of white matter integrity in bipolar disorder. *Epidemiol Psychiatr Sci.* 2011;20:137-140.

Beltz BS, Tlusty MF, Benton JL, and Sandeman DC. Omega-3 fatty acids upregulate adult neurogenesis. *Neurosci Lett.* 2007;415:154-158.

Bhutta AT, Cleves MA, Casey PH, Cradock MM, and Anand KJ. Cognitive and behavioral outcomes of school-aged children who were born preterm: a meta-analysis. *JAMA.* 2002;288:728-737.

Bloch MH and Qawasmi A. Omega-3 fatty acid supplementation for the treatment of children with attention-deficit/hyperactivity disorder symptomatology: systematic review and meta-analysis. *J Am Acad Child Adolesc Psychiatry.* 2011;50:991-1000.

Blondeau N, Widmann C, Lazdunski M, and Heurteaux C. Polyunsaturated fatty acids induce ischemic and epileptic tolerance. *Neuroscience.* 2002;109:231-241.

Bondi CO, Taha AY, Tock JL, Totah NK, Cheon Y, Torres GE, Rapoport SI, and Moghaddam B. Adolescent behavior and dopamine availability are uniquely sensitive to dietary omega-3 fatty acid deficiency. *Biol Psychiatry*. 2014;75:38-46.

Bora E, Fornito A, Pantelis C, and Yücel M. Gray matter abnormalities in major depressive disorder: a meta-analysis of voxel based morphometry studies. J *Affect Disord*. 2012;138:9-18.

Botting N, Powls A, Cooke RW, and Marlow N. Attention deficit hyperactivity disorders and other psychiatric outcomes in very low birthweight children at 12 years. *J Child Psychol Psychiatry*. 1997;38:931-941.

Boucher O, Burden MJ, Muckle G, Saint-Amour D, Ayotte P, Dewailly E, Nelson CA, Jacobson SW, and Jacobson JL. Neurophysiologic and neurobehavioral evidence of beneficial effects of prenatal omega-3 fatty acid intake on memory function at school age. *Am J Clin Nutr*. 2011;93:1025-1037.

Brand, A., C. Richter-Landsberg, and D. and Leibfritz. Multinuclear NMR studies on the energy metabolism of glial and neuronal cells. *Dev. Neurosci.* 1993;15:289-298.

Brenna JT, Salem N Jr, Sinclair AJ, Cunnane SC, and International Society for the Study of Fatty Acids and Lipids, ISSFAL. alpha-Linolenic acid supplementation and conversion to *n*-3 long-chain polyunsaturated fatty acids in humans. *Prostaglandins Leukot Essent Fatty Acids*. 2009;80:85-91.

Brenna JT, Varamini B, Jensen RG, Diersen-Schade DA, Boettcher JA, and Arterburn LM. Docosahexaenoic and arachidonic acid concentrations in human breast milk worldwide. *Am J Clin Nutr*. 2007;85:1457-1464.

Brown S. Excess mortality of schizophrenia. A meta-analysis. *Br J Psychiatry*. 1997;171:502-508.

Burdge GC and Wootton SA. Conversion of alpha-linolenic acid to eicosapentaenoic, docosapentaenoic and docosahexaenoic acids in young women. *Br J Nutr*. 2002;88:411-420.

Burke KC, Burke JD Jr, Rae DS, and Regier DA. Comparing age at onset of major depression and other psychiatric disorders by birth cohorts in five US community populations. *Arch Gen Psychiatry*. 1991;48:789-795.

Byard RW, Makrides M, Need M, Neumann MA, and Gibson RA. Sudden infant death syndrome: effect of breast and formula feeding on frontal cortex and brainstem lipid composition. *J Paediatr Child Health*. 1995;31:14-16.

Calderon F and Kim HY. Docosahexaenoic acid promotes neurite growth in hippocampal neurons. *J Neurochem*. 2004;90:979-988.

Calon F and Cole G. Neuroprotective action of omega-3 polyunsaturated fatty acids against neurodegenerative diseases: evidence from animal studies. Prostaglandins Leukot Essent Fatty Acids. 2007;77:287-293.

Canu E, Agosta F, and Filippi M. A selective review of structural connectivity abnormalities of schizophrenic patients at different stages of the disease. *Schizophr Res*. 2014 [Epub ahead of print]

Cao D, Kevala K, Kim J, Moon HS, Jun SB, Lovinger D, and Kim HY. Docosahexaenoic acid promotes hippocampal neuronal development and synaptic function. *J Neurochem*. 2009;111:510-521.

Cao X, Cao Q, Long X, Sun L, Sui M, Zhu C, Zuo X, Zang Y, and Wang Y. Abnormal resting-state functional connectivity patterns of the putamen in medication-naïve children with attention deficit hyperactivity disorder. *Brain Res*. 2009;1303:195-206.

Carlezon WA Jr, Mague SD, Parow AM, Stoll AL, Cohen BM, and Renshaw PF. Antidepressant-like effects of uridine and omega-3 fatty acids are potentiated by combined treatment in rats. *Biol Psychiatry*. 2005;57:343-350.

Carlson SE, Colombo J, Gajewski BJ, Gustafson KM, Mundy D, Yeast J, Georgieff MK, Markley LA, Kerling EH, and Shaddy DJ. DHA supplementation and pregnancy outcomes. *The American journal of clinical nutrition* 2013;97:808-815.

Carlson SE, Rhodes PG, and Ferguson MG. Docosahexaenoic acid status of preterm infants at birth and following feeding with human milk or formula. Am *J Clin Nutr*. 1986;44:798-804.

Carlson SE. Docosahexaenoic acid supplementation in pregnancy and lactation. *Am J Clin Nutr*. 2009;89:678S-684S.

Carrié I, Smirnova M, Clément M, DE JD, Francès H, and Bourre JM. Docosahexaenoic acid-rich phospholipid supplementation: effect on behavior, learning ability, and retinal function in control and *n*-3 polyunsaturated fatty acid deficient old mice. *Nutr Neurosci*. 2002;5:43-52.

Carver JD, Benford VJ, Han B, and Cantor AB. The relationship between age and the fatty acid composition of cerebral cortex and erythrocytes in human subjects. *Brain Res Bull*. 2001;56:79-85.

Castellanos FX, Lee PP, Sharp W, Jeffries NO, Greenstein DK, Clasen LS, Blumenthal JD, James RS, Ebens CL, Walter JM, Zijdenbos A, Evans AC, Giedd JN, and Rapoport JL. Developmental trajectories of brain volume abnormalities in children and adolescents with attention-deficit/hyperactivity disorder. *JAMA*. 2002;288:1740-1748.

Cavanagh J, Smyth R, and Goodwin GM. Relapse into mania or depression following lithium discontinuation: a 7-year follow-up. Acta Psychiatr Scand. 2004;109:91-95.

Chalon S, Delion-Vancassel S, Belzung C, Guilloteau D, Leguisquet AM, Besnard JC, and Durand G. Dietary fish oil affects monoaminergic neurotransmission and behavior in rats. *J Nutr*. 1998;128:2512-2519.

Cheatham CL, Nerhammer AS, Asserhøj M, Michaelsen KF, and Lauritzen L. Fish oil supplementation during lactation: effects on cognition and behavior at 7 years of age. *Lipids*. 2011;46:637-645.

Chen CT, Liu Z, Ouellet M, Calon F, and Bazinet RP. Rapid beta-oxidation of eicosapentaenoic acid in mouse brain: an in situ study. *Prostaglandins Leukot Essent Fatty Acids*. 2009;80:157-163.

Cheruku SR, Montgomery-Downs HE, Farkas SL, Thoman EB, and Lammi-Keefe CJ. Higher maternal plasma docosahexaenoic acid during pregnancy is associated with more mature neonatal sleep-state patterning. *Am J Clin Nutr*. 2002;76:608-613.

Chiu CC, Huang SY, Su KP, Lu ML, Huang MC, Chen CC, and Shen WW. Polyunsaturated fatty acid deficit in patients with bipolar mania. *Eur Neuropsychopharmacol*. 2003;13:99-103.

Chuang TC, Wu MT, Huang SP, Weng MJ, and Yang P. Diffusion tensor imaging study of white matter fiber tracts in adolescent attention-deficit/hyperactivity disorder. *Psychiatry Res*. 2013;211:186-187.

Clandinin MT, Chappell JE, Leong S, Heim T, Swyer PR, and Chance GW. Intrauterine fatty acid accretion rates in human brain: implications for fatty acid requirements. *Early Hum Dev*. 1980a;4:121-129.

Clandinin MT, Chappell JE, Leong S, Heim T, Swyer PR, and Chance GW. Extrauterine fatty acid accretion in infant brain: implications for fatty acid requirements. *Early Hum Dev*. 1980b;4:131-138.

Clayton EH, Hanstock TL, Hirneth SJ, Kable CJ, Garg ML, and Hazell PL. Long-chain omega-3 polyunsaturated fatty acids in the blood of children and adolescents with juvenile bipolar disorder. *Lipids*. 2008;43:1031-1038.

Clayton EH, Hanstock TL, Hirneth SJ, Kable CJ, Garg ML, and Hazell PL. Reduced mania and depression in juvenile bipolar disorder associated with long-chain omega-3 polyunsaturated fatty acid supplementation. *Eur J Clin Nutr*. 2009;63:1037-1040.

Clayton EH, Hanstock TL, and Watson JF. Estimated intakes of meat and fish by children and adolescents in Australia and comparison with recommendations. *Br J Nutr*. 2009a;101:1731-1735.

Coccaro EF, Kavoussi RJ, Trestman RL, Gabriel SM, Cooper TB, and Siever LJ. Serotonin function in human subjects: intercorrelations among central 5-HT indices and aggressiveness. *Psychiatry Res*. 1997;73:1-14.

Colangelo LA, He K, Whooley MA, Daviglus ML, and Liu K. Higher dietary intake of long-chain omega-3 polyunsaturated fatty acids is inversely associated with depressive symptoms in women. *Nutrition*. 2009;25:1011-1019.

Colombo J, Kannass KN, Shaddy DJ, Kundurthi S, Maikranz JM, Anderson CJ, Blaga OM, Carlson SE. Maternal DHA, and the development of attention in infancy and toddlerhood. *Child Dev*. 2004;75:1254-1267.

Colombo RR, Schaufelberger MS, Santos LC, Duran FL, Menezes PR, Scazufca M, Busatto GF, and Zanetti MV. Voxelwise evaluation of white matter volumes in first-episode psychosis. *Psychiatry Res*. 2012;202:198-205.

Conklin HM, Luciana M, Hooper CJ, and Yarger RS. Working memory performance in typically developing children and adolescents: behavioral evidence of protracted frontal lobe development. *Dev Neuropsychol*. 2007;31:103-128.

Conklin SM, Runyan CA, Leonard S, Reddy RD, Muldoon MF, and Yao JK. Age-related changes of *n*-3 and *n*-6 polyunsaturated fatty acids in the anterior cingulate cortex of individuals with major depressive disorder. *Prostaglandins Leukot Essent Fatty Acids*. 2010;82:111-119.

Connor WE, Neuringer M, and Lin DS. Dietary effects on brain fatty acid composition: the reversibility of *n*-3 fatty acid deficiency and turnover of docosahexaenoic acid in the brain, erythrocytes, and plasma of rhesus monkeys. *J Lipid Res*. 1990;31:237-247.

Constable RT, Ment LR, Vohr BR, Kesler SR, Fulbright RK, Lacadie C, Delancy S, Katz KH, Schneider KC, Schafer RJ, Makuch RW, and Reiss AR. Prematurely born children demonstrate white matter microstructural differences at 12 years of age, relative to term control subjects: an investigation of group and gender effects. *Pediatrics*. 2008;121:306-316.

Conus P, Ward J, Hallam KT, Lucas N, Macneil C, McGorry PD, and Berk M. The proximal prodrome to first episode mania--a new target for early intervention. *Bipolar Disord*. 2008;10:555-565.

Cooke RW and Foulder-Hughes L. Growth impairment in the very preterm and cognitive and motor performance at 7 years. Arch Dis Child. 2003;88:482-487.

Coti Bertrand P, O'Kusky JR, and Innis SM. Maternal dietary (*n*-3) fatty acid deficiency alters neurogenesis in the embryonic rat brain. J Nutr. 2006;136:1570-1575.

Cullen KR, Klimes-Dougan B, Muetzel R, Mueller BA, Camchong J, Houri A, Kurma S, and Lim KO. Altered white matter microstructure in adolescents with major depression: a preliminary study. *J Am Acad Child Adolesc Psychiatry*. 2010;49:173-183.

De Peri L, Crescini A, Deste G, Fusar-Poli P, Sacchetti E, and Vita A. Brain structural abnormalities at the onset of schizophrenia and bipolar disorder: a meta-analysis of controlled magnetic resonance imaging studies. *Curr Pharm Des*. 2012;18:486-494.

Delion S, Chalon S, Guilloteau D, Besnard JC, and Durand G. alpha-Linolenic acid dietary deficiency alters age-related changes of dopaminergic and serotoninergic neurotransmission in the rat frontal cortex. *J Neurochem*. 1996;66:1582-1591.

DeMar JC Jr, Ma K, Bell JM, Igarashi M, Greenstein D, and Rapoport SI. One generation of *n*-3 polyunsaturated fatty acid deprivation increases depression and aggression test scores in rats. *J Lipid Res*. 2006;47:172-180.

DeMar JC Jr, Ma K, Bell JM, and Rapoport SI. Half-lives of docosahexaenoic acid in rat brain phospholipids are prolonged by 15 weeks of nutritional deprivation of *n*-3 polyunsaturated fatty acids. *J. Neurochem*. 2004;91:1125-1137.

Diau GY, Loew ER, Wijendran V, Sarkadi-Nagy E, Nathanielsz PW, and Brenna JT. Docosahexaenoic and arachidonic acid influence on preterm baboon retinal composition and function. *Invest Ophthalmol Vis Sci*. 2003;44:4559-4566.

Dickstein DP, Gorrostieta C, Ombao H, Goldberg LD, Brazel AC, Gable CJ, Kelly C, Gee DG, Zuo XN, Castellanos FX, and Milham MP. Fronto-temporal spontaneous resting state functional connectivity in pediatric bipolar disorder. *Biol Psychiatry*. 2010;68:839-846.

Dobbing J and Sands J. Quantitative growth and development of human brain. Arch Dis Child. 1973;48:757-767.

Ducharme S, Hudziak JJ, Botteron KN, Albaugh MD, Nguyen TV, Karama S, Evans AC, and Brain Development Cooperative Group. Decreased regional cortical thickness and thinning rate are associated with inattention symptoms in healthy children. *J Am Acad Child Adolesc Psychiatry.* 2012;51:18-27.

Dutta-Roy AK. Transport mechanisms for long-chain polyunsaturated fatty acids in the human placenta. *Am J Clin Nutr.* 2000;71:315S-322S.

Dyall SC, Michael GJ, Whelpton R, Scott AG, and Michael-Titus AT. Dietary enrichment with omega-3 polyunsaturated fatty acids reverses age-related decreases in the GluR2 and NR2B glutamate receptor subunits in rat forebrain. *Neurobiol Aging.* 2007;28:424-439.

Ebeling U and von Cramon D. Topography of the uncinate fascicle and adjacent temporal fiber tracts. *Acta Neurochir* (Wien). 1992;115:143-148.

Ehringer MA, Rhee SH, Young S, Corley R, and Hewitt JK. Genetic and environmental contributions to common psychopathologies of childhood and adolescence: a study of twins and their siblings. *J. Abnorm. Child. Psychol.* 2006;34:1-17.

Emsley R, Myburgh C, Oosthuizen P, van and Rensburg SJ. Randomized, placebo-controlled study of ethyl-eicosapentaenoic acid as supplemental treatment in schizophrenia. *Am. J. Psychiatry.* 2002;159:1596-1598.

Ernst M, Zametkin AJ, Matochik JA, Jons PH, and Cohen RM. DOPA decarboxylase activity in attention deficit hyperactivity disorder adults. A [fluorine-18]fluorodopa positron emission tomographic study. *J. Neurosci.* 1998;18:5901-5907.

Farooqui AA and Horrocks LA. Brain phospholipases A2: a perspective on the history. *Prostaglandins Leukot Essent Fatty Acids* 2004;71:161-169.

Farquharson J, Cockburn F, Patrick WA, Jamieson EC, and Logan RW. Infant cerebral cortex phospholipid fatty-acid composition and diet. *Lancet.* 1992;340:810-813.

Farquharson J, Jamieson EC, Abbasi KA, Patrick WJ, Logan RW, and Cockburn F. Effect of diet on the fatty acid composition of the major phospholipids of infant cerebral cortex. *Arch Dis Child.* 1995;72:198-203.

Fedorova I, Alvheim AR, Hussein N, and Salem N Jr. Deficit in prepulse inhibition in mice caused by dietary *n*-3 fatty acid deficiency. *Behav Neurosci.* 2009;123:1218-1225.

Fedorova I, Hussein N, Baumann MH, Di Martino C, and Salem N Jr. An *n*-3 fatty acid deficiency impairs rat spatial learning in the Barnes maze. *Behav Neurosci.* 2009;123:196-205.

Fekete K, Marosvölgyi T, Jakobik V, and Decsi T. Methods of assessment of *n*-3 long-chain polyunsaturated fatty acid status in humans: a systematic review. *Am J Clin Nutr.* 2009;89:2070S-2084S.

Flock MR, Skulas-Ray AC, Harris WS, Etherton TD, Fleming JA, and Kris-Etherton PM. Determinants of erythrocyte omega-3 fatty acid content in response to fish oil supplementation: a dose-response randomized controlled trial. *J Am Heart Assoc*. 2013;2:e000513.

Foulder-Hughes LA and Cooke RW. Motor, cognitive, and behavioural disorders in children born very preterm. *Dev Med Child Neurol*. 2003;4:97-103.

Francois CA, Connor SL, Bolewicz LC, and Connor WE. Supplementing lactating women with flaxseed oil does not increase docosahexaenoic acid in their milk. *Am J Clin Nutr*. 2003;77:226-233.

Frangou S, Lewis M, Wollard J, and Simmons A. Preliminary in vivo evidence of increased *N*-acetyl-aspartate following eicosapentanoic acid treatment in patients with bipolar disorder. *J Psychopharmacol*. 2007;21:435-439.

Fujita S, Ikegaya Y, Nishikawa M, Nishiyama N, and Matsuki N. Docosahexaenoic acid improves long-term potentiation attenuated by phospholipase A(2) inhibitor in rat hippocampal slices. *Br J Pharmacol*. 2001;132:1417-1422.

Gama CS, Canever L, Panizzutti B, Gubert C, Stertz L, Massuda R, Pedrini M, de Lucena DF, Luca RD, Fraga DB, Heylmann AS, Deroza PF, and Zugno AI. Effects of omega-3 dietary supplement in prevention of positive, negative and cognitive symptoms: a study in adolescent rats with ketamine-induced model of schizophrenia. *Schizophr Res*. 2012;141:162-167.

Geddes JR, Carney SM, Davies C, Furukawa TA, Kupfer DJ, Frank E, and Goodwin GM. Relapse prevention with antidepressant drug treatment in depressive disorders: a systematic review. *Lancet* 2003;361:653-661.

Gibson RA, Neumann MA, and Makrides M. Effect of dietary docosahexaenoic acid on brain composition and neural function in term infants. *Lipids*. 1996;31:S177-181.

Giedd JN, Lalonde FM, Celano MJ, White SL, Wallace GL, Lee NR, and Lenroot RK. Anatomical brain magnetic resonance imaging of typically developing children and adolescents. *J Am Acad Child Adolesc Psychiatry*. 2009;48:465-470.

Glahn DC, Laird AR, Ellison-Wright I, Thelen SM, Robinson JL, Lancaster JL, Bullmore E, and Fox PT. Meta-analysis of gray matter anomalies in schizophrenia: application of anatomic likelihood estimation and network analysis. *Biol Psychiatry*. 2008;64:774-781.

Glantz LA, Gilmore JH, Hamer RM, Lieberman JA, and Jarskog LF. Synaptophysin and postsynaptic density protein 95 in the human prefrontal cortex from mid-gestation into early adulthood. *Neuroscience*. 2007;149:582-591.

Gozzo Y, Vohr B, Lacadie C, Hampson M, Katz KH, Maller-Kesselman J, Schneider KC, Peterson BS, Rajeevan N, Makuch RW, Constable RT, and Ment LR. Alterations in neural connectivity in preterm children at school age. *Neuroimage*. 2009;48:458-463.

Grayson DS, Kroenke CD, Neuringer M, and Fair DA. Dietary omega-3 fatty acids modulate large-scale systems organization in the rhesus macaque brain. *J Neurosci*. 2014;34:2065-2074.

Green P, Glozman S, Weiner L, and Yavin E. Enhanced free radical scavenging and decreased lipid peroxidation in the rat fetal brain after treatment with ethyl docosahexaenoate. *Biochim Biophys Acta*. 2001;1532:203-212.

Green P and Yavin E. Fatty acid composition of late embryonic and early postnatal rat brain. *Lipids*. 1996;31:859-865.

Greenberg PE, Kessler RC, Birnbaum HG, Leong SA, Lowe SW, Berglund PA, and Corey-Lisle PK. The economic burden of depression in the United States: how did it change between 1990 and 2000? *J Clin Psychiatry*. 2003;64:1465-1475.

Greiner RS, Moriguchi T, Hutton A, Slotnick BM, and Salem N Jr. Rats with low levels of brain docosahexaenoic acid show impaired performance in olfactory-based and spatial learning tasks. *Lipids*. 1999;34 Suppl:S239-43.

Greiner RS, Moriguchi T, Slotnick BM, Hutton A, and Salem N. Olfactory discrimination deficits in *n*-3 fatty acid-deficient rats. *Physiol Behav*. 2001;72:379-385.

Griffin, J. L., M. Bollard, J. K. Nicholson, and K. Bhakoo. Spectral profiles of cultured neuronal and glial cells derived from HRMAS (1)H NMR spectroscopy. *NMR Biomed*. 2002;15:375-384.

Grosso G, Pajak A, Marventano S, Castellano S, Galvano F, Bucolo C, Drago F, and Caraci F. Role of omega-3 fatty acids in the treatment of depressive disorders: a comprehensive meta-analysis of randomized clinical trials. *PLoS One*. 2014;9:e96905.

Guo WB, Liu F, Xue ZM, Gao K, Wu RR, Ma CQ, Liu ZN, Xiao CQ, Chen HF, and Zhao JP. Altered white matter integrity in young adults with first-episode, treatment-naive, and treatment-responsive depression. *Neurosci Lett*. 2012;522: 139-144.

Harel Z, Riggs S, Vaz R, White L, and Menzies G. Omega-3 polyunsaturated fatty acids in adolescents: knowledge and consumption. *J Adolesc Health*. 2001;28:10-15.

Hawkey E and Nigg JT. Omega-3 fatty acid and ADHD: Blood level analysis and meta-analytic extension of supplementation trials. *Clin Psychol Rev.* 2014 [Epub ahead of print].

Helland IB, Smith L, Blomén B, Saarem K, Saugstad OD, and Drevon CA. Effect of supplementing pregnant and lactating mothers with *n*-3 very-long-chain fatty acids on children's IQ and body mass index at 7 years of age. *Pediatrics.* 2008;122:472-479.

Helland IB, Smith L, Saarem K, Saugstad OD, and Drevon CA. Maternal supplementation with very-long-chain *n*-3 fatty acids during pregnancy and lactation augments children's IQ at 4 years of age. *Pediatrics.* 2003;111:e39-44.

Hibbeln JR, Davis JM, Steer C, Emmett P, Rogers I, Williams C, and Golding J. Maternal seafood consumption in pregnancy and neurodevelopmental outcomes in childhood (ALSPAC study): an observational cohort study. *Lancet.* 2007;369:578-585.

Hibbeln JR. Fish consumption and major depression. *Lancet* 1998;351:1213.

Hichami A, Datiche F, Ullah S, Liénard F, Chardigny JM, Cattarelli M, and Khan NA. Olfactory discrimination ability and brain expression of c-fos, Gir and Glut1 mRNA are altered in *n*-3 fatty acid-depleted rats. *Behav Brain Res.* 2007;184:1-10.

Hoen WP, Lijmer JG, Duran M, Wanders RJ, van Beveren NJ, and de Haan L. Red blood cell polyunsaturated fatty acids measured in red blood cells and schizophrenia: A meta-analysis. *Psychiatry Res.* 2013;207:1-12.

Högyes E, Nyakas C, Kiliaan A, Farkas T, Penke B, and Luiten PG. Neuroprotective effect of developmental docosahexaenoic acid supplement against excitotoxic brain damage in infant rats. *Neuroscience.* 2003;119:999-1012.

Huang SY, Yang HT, Chiu CC, Pariante CM, and Su KP. Omega-3 fatty acids on the forced-swimming test. *J Psychiatr Res.* 2008;42:58-63.

Huttenlocher PR. Synaptic density in human frontal cortex - developmental changes and effects of aging. *Brain Res.* 1979;163:195-205.

Igarashi M, Ma K, Gao F, and Kim HW, Greenstein D, Rapoport SI, Rao JS. Brain lipid concentrations in bipolar disorder. *J Psychiatr Res.* 2010;44:177-182.

Ikemoto A, Kobayashi T, Watanabe S, and Okuyama H. Membrane fatty acid modifications of PC12 cells by arachidonate or docosahexaenoate affect neurite outgrowth but not norepinephrine release. *Neurochem Res.* 1997;22:671-678.

Ikemoto A, Nitta A, Furukawa S, Ohishi M, Nakamura A, Fujii Y, and Okuyama H. Dietary *n*-3 fatty acid deficiency decreases nerve growth factor content in rat hippocampus. *Neurosci Lett.* 2000;285:99-102.

Innis SM, Gilley J and Werker J. Are human milk long-chain polyunsaturated fatty acids related to visual and neural development in breast-fed term infants? *J Pediatr.* 2001b;139:532-538.

Itokazu N, Ikegaya Y, Nishikawa M, and Matsuki N. Bidirectional actions of docosahexaenoic acid on hippocampal neurotransmissions in vivo. Brain Res. 2000;862:211-216.

Itomura M, Fujioka S, Hamazaki K, Kobayashi K, Nagasawa T, Sawazaki S, Kirihara Y, and Hamazaki T. Factors influencing EPA+DHA levels in red blood cells in Japan. In Vivo. 2008;22:131-135.

Jacques C, Levy E, Muckle G, Jacobson SW, Bastien C, Dewailly E, Ayotte P, Jacobson JL, and Saint-Amour D. Long-term effects of prenatal omega-3 fatty acid intake on visual function in school-age children. *J Pediatr.* 2011;158:83-90.

Jamieson EC, Farquharson J, Logan RW, Howatson AG, Patrick WJ, Weaver LT, and Cockburn F. Infant cerebellar gray and white matter fatty acids in relation to age and diet. *Lipids.* 1999;34:1065-1071.

Jensen CL, Maude M, Anderson RE, and Heird WC. Effect of docosahexaenoic acid supplementation of lactating women on the fatty acid composition of breast milk lipids and maternal and infant plasma phospholipids. *Am J Clin Nutr.* 2000;71:292S-299S.

Johnson S, Hollis C, Kochhar P, Hennessy E, Wolke D, and Marlow N. Psychiatric disorders in extremely preterm children: longitudinal finding at age 11 years in the EPICure study. *J Am Acad Child Adolesc Psychiatry.* 2010;49:453-463.

Kawakita E, Hashimoto M, and Shido O. Docosahexaenoic acid promotes neurogenesis in vitro and in vivo. *Neuroscience.* 2006;139:991-997.

Keleshian VL, Kellom M, Kim HW, Taha AY, Cheon Y, Igarashi M, Rapoport SI, and Rao JS. Neuropathological responses to chronic NMDA in rats are worsened by dietary *n*-3 PUFA deprivation but are not ameliorated by fish oil supplementation. *PLoS One.* 2014;9:e95318.

Kempton MJ, Salvador Z, Munafò MR, Geddes JR, Simmons A, Frangou S, and Williams SC. Structural neuroimaging studies in major depressive disorder. Meta-analysis and comparison with bipolar disorder. *Arch Gen Psychiatry.* 2011;68:675-690.

Kesler SR, Reiss AL, Vohr B, Watson C, Schneider KC, Katz KH, Maller-Kesselman J, Silbereis J, Constable RT, Makuch RW, and Ment LR. Brain volume reductions within multiple cognitive systems in male preterm children at age twelve. *J Pediatr*. 2008;152:513-520.

Kessler RC, Berglund P, Demler O, Jin R, Merikangas KR, and Walters EE. Lifetime prevalence and age-of-onset distributions of DSM-IV disorders in the National Comorbidity Survey Replication. *Arch Gen Psychiatry*. 2005;62:593-602.

Kessler RC, Merikangas KR, and Wang PS. Prevalence, comorbidity, and service utilization for mood disorders in the United States at the beginning of the twenty-first century. *Annu Rev Clin Psychol*. 2007;3:137-158.

Khan MM, Evans DR, Gunna V, Scheffer RE, Parikh VV, and Mahadik SP. Reduced erythrocyte membrane essential fatty acids and increased lipid peroxides in schizophrenia at the never-medicated first-episode of psychosis and after years of treatment with antipsychotics. *Schizophr. Res*. 2002;58:1-10.

Kier EL, Staib LH, Davis LM, and Bronen RA. MR imaging of the temporal stem: anatomic dissection tractography of the uncinate fasciculus, inferior occipitofrontal fasciculus, and Meyer's loop of the optic radiation. *AJNR Am J Neuroradiol*. 2004;25:677-691.

Kirby A, Woodward A, Jackson S, Wang Y, and Crawford MA. A double-blind, placebo-controlled study investigating the effects of omega-3 supplementation in children aged 8-10 years from a mainstream school population. *Res Dev Disabil*. 2010;31:718-730.

Kleinman L, Lowin A, Flood E, Gandhi G, Edgell E, and Revicki D. Costs of bipolar disorder. *Pharmacoeconomics*. 2003;21:601-622.

Kodas E, Page G, Zimmer L, Vancassel S, Guilloteau D, Durand G, and Chalon S. Neither the density nor function of striatal dopamine transporters were influenced by chronic *n*-3 polyunsaturated fatty acid deficiency in rodents. *Neurosci Lett*. 2002b;321:95-99.

Kodas E, Vancassel S, Lejeune B, Guilloteau D, and Chalon S. Reversibility of *n*-3 fatty acid deficiency-induced changes in dopaminergic neurotransmission in rats: critical role of developmental stage. *J Lipid Res*. 2002a;43:1209-1219.

Kodas E, Galineau L, Bodard S, Vancassel S, Guilloteau D, Besnard JC, and Chalon S. Serotoninergic neurotransmission is affected by *n*-3 polyunsaturated fatty acids in the rat. *J Neurochem*. 2004;89:695-702.

Kohlboeck G, Glaser C, Tiesler C, Demmelmair H, Standl M, Romanos M, Koletzko B, Lehmann I, Heinrich J, and LISAplus Study Group. Effect of fatty acid status in cord blood serum on children's behavioral difficulties at

10 y of age: results from the LISAplus Study. *Am J Clin Nutr.* 2011;94:1592-1599.

Koletzko B, Larqué E, and Demmelmair H. Placental transfer of long-chain polyunsaturated fatty acids (LC-PUFA). *J Perinat Med.* 2007;35:S5-11.

Koletzko B, Lattka E, Zeilinger S, Illig T, and Steer C. Genetic variants of the fatty acid desaturase gene cluster predict amounts of red blood cell docosahexaenoic and other polyunsaturated fatty acids in pregnant women: findings from the Avon Longitudinal Study of Parents and Children. *Am J Clin Nutr.* 2011;93:211-219.

Krabbendam L, Bakker E, Hornstra G, and van Os J. Relationship between DHA status at birth and child problem behaviour at 7 years of age. *Prostaglandins Leukot Essent Fatty Acids.* 2007;76:29-34.

Kuperstein F, Eilam R, and Yavin E. Altered expression of key dopaminergic regulatory proteins in the postnatal brain following perinatal *n*-3 fatty acid dietary deficiency. *J Neurochem.* 2008;106:662-671.

Laino CH, Fonseca C, Sterin-Speziale N, Slobodianik N, and Reinés A. Potentiation of omega-3 fatty acid antidepressant-like effects with low non-antidepressant doses of fluoxetine and mirtazapine. *Eur J Pharmacol.* 2010;648:117-126.

Lakhwani L, Tongia SK, Pal VS, Agrawal RP, Nyati P, and Phadnis P. Omega-3 fatty acids have antidepressant activity in forced swimming test in Wistar rats. *Acta Pol Pharm.* 2007;64:271-276.

Lalovic A, Levy E, Canetti L, Sequeira A, Montoudis A, and Turecki G. Fatty acid composition in postmortem brains of people who completed suicide. *J Psychiatry Neurosci.* 2007;32:363-370.

Lanfermann H, Kugel H, Heindel W, Herholz K, Heiss WD, and Lackner K. Metabolic changes in acute and subacute cerebral infarctions: findings at proton MR spectroscopic imaging. *Radiology.* 1995;196:203-210.

Lauritzen L, Jørgensen MH, Hansen HS, and Michaelsen KF. Fluctuations in human milk long-chain PUFA levels in relation to dietary fish intake. *Lipids.* 2002;37:237-244.

Lauritzen L, Harsløf LB, Hellgren LI, Pedersen MH, Mølgaard C, and Michaelsen KF. Fish intake, erythrocyte *n*-3 fatty acid status and metabolic health in Danish adolescent girls and boys. *Br J Nutr.* 2012;107:697-704.

Lawrence KE, Levitt JG, Loo SK, Ly R, Yee V, O'Neill J, Alger J, and Narr KL. White matter microstructure in subjects with attention-deficit/hyperactivity disorder and their siblings. *J Am Acad Child Adolesc Psychiatry.* 2013;52:431-440.

Levant B, Radel JD, and Carlson SE. Decreased brain docosahexaenoic acid during development alters dopamine-related behaviors in adult rats that are differentially affected by dietary remediation. *Behav Brain Res.* 2004;152:49-57.

Lin PY, Huang SY, and Su KP. A meta-analytic review of polyunsaturated fatty acid compositions in patients with depression. *Biol Psychiatry.* 2010;68:140-147.

Lin YH, Shah S, and Salem N Jr. Altered essential fatty acid metabolism and composition in rat liver, plasma, heart and brain after microalgal DHA addition to the diet. *J Nutr Biochem.* 2011a;22:758-765.

Lin F, Weng S, Xie B, Wu G, and Lei H. Abnormal frontal cortex white matter connections in bipolar disorder: a DTI tractography study. *J Affect Disord.* 2011b;131:299-306.

Lotrich FE, Sears B, and McNamara RK. Elevated ratio of arachidonic acid to long-chain omega-3 fatty acids predicts depression development following interferon-alpha treatment: Relationship with interleukin-6. Brain Behav Immun. 2013;31:48-53.

Lubsen J, Vohr B, Myers E, Hampson M, Lacadie C, Schneider KC, and Katz KH, Constable RT, Ment LR. Microstructural and functional connectivity in the developing preterm brain. *Semin Perinatol.* 2011;35:34-43.

Makrides M, Gibson RA, McPhee AJ, Yelland L, Quinlivan J, Ryan P, and DOMInO Investigative Team. Effect of DHA supplementation during pregnancy on maternal depression and neurodevelopment of young children: a randomized controlled trial. *JAMA.* 2010;304:1675-1683.

Makrides M, Gould JF, Gawlik NR, Yelland LN, Smithers LG, Anderson PJ, and Gibson RA. Four-year follow-up of children born to women in a randomized trial of prenatal DHA supplementation. *JAMA.* 2014;311:1802-1804.

Makrides M, Neumann MA, Byard RW, Simmer K, and Gibson RA. Fatty acid composition of brain, retina, and erythrocytes in breast- and formula-fed infants. *Am J Clin Nutr.* 1994;60:189-194.

Mansbach RS, Geyer MA, and Braff DL. Dopaminergic stimulation disrupts sensorimotor gating in the rat. *Psychopharmacology (Berl).* 1988;94:507-514.

Martin DS, Spencer P, Horrobin DF, and Lynch MA. Long-term potentiation in aged rats is restored when the age-related decrease in polyunsaturated fatty acid concentration is reversed. *Prostaglandins Leukot Essent Fatty Acids.* 2002;67:121-130.

Martínez M and Mougan I. Fatty acid composition of human brain phospholipids during normal development. *J Neurochem.* 1998;71:2528-2533.

Martinez M. Abnormal profiles of polyunsaturated fatty acids in the brain, liver, kidney and retina of patients with peroxisomal disorders. *Brain Res.* 1992;583:171-182.

Martinez M. Tissue levels of polyunsaturated fatty acids during early human development. *J Pediatr.* 1992;120:S129-138.

McGahon BM, Martin DS, Horrobin DF, and Lynch MA. Age-related changes in synaptic function: analysis of the effect of dietary supplementation with omega-3 fatty acids. Neuroscience. 1999;94:305-314.

McGuffin P, Owen MJ, and Gottesman II., Eds Psychiatric Genetics and Genomics (revised) Oxford: Oxford University Press; 2004.

McNamara RK, Ostrander M, Abplanalp W, Richtand NM, Benoit SC, and Clegg DJ. Modulation of phosphoinositide-protein kinase C signal transduction by omega-3 fatty acids: implications for the pathophysiology and treatment of recurrent neuropsychiatric illness. *Prostaglandins Leukot Essent Fatty Acids.* 2006;75:237-257.

McNamara RK, Hahn C-G, Jandacek R, Rider T, Tso P, Stanford K, and Richtand NM. Selective deficits in the omega-3 fatty acid docosahexaenoic acid in the postmortem orbitofrontal cortex of patients with major depressive disorder. *Biol Psychiatry* 2007a;62:17-24.

McNamara RK, Jandacek R, Rider T, Tso P, Richtand NM, and Stanford K. Abnormalities in the fatty acid composition of the postmortem orbitofrontal cortex of schizophrenic patients: Gender differences and partial normalization with antipsychotic medications. *Schizophr Res.* 2007b;91:37-50.

McNamara RK, Liu Y, Jandacek R, Rider T, and Tso P. The aging human orbitofrontal cortex: Decreasing polyunsaturated fatty acid composition and associated increases in lipogenic gene expression and stearoyl-CoA desaturase activity. *Prostaglandins Leukot Essent Fatty Acids 2008a*;78:293-304.

McNamara RK, Jandacek R, Rider T, Tso P, Stanford K, Hahn C-G, and Richtand NM. Deficits in docosahexaenoic acid and associated elevations in the metabolism of arachidonic acid and saturated fatty acids in the postmortem orbitofrontal cortex of patients with bipolar disorder. *Psychiatric Res.* 2008b;160:285-299.

McNamara RK, Sullivan J, and Richtand NM. Omega-3 fatty acid deficiency augments amphetamine-induced behavioral sensitization in adult mice:

Prevention by chronic lithium treatment. *J Psychiatric Res*. 2008c;42:458-468.

McNamara RK, Sullivan J, Richtand NM, Jandacek R, Rider T, Tso P, Campbell N, and Lipton JW. Omega-3 fatty acid deficiency augments amphetamine-induced behavioral sensitization in adult DBA/2J mice: Relationship with ventral striatum dopamine concentrations. *Synapse* 2008d;62:725-735.

McNamara RK, Able J, Liu Y, Jandacek R, Rider T, Tso P, and Lipton JW. Omega-3 fatty acid deficiency during perinatal development increases serotonin turnover in the prefrontal cortex and decreases midbrain tryptophan hydroxylase-2 expression in adult female rats: dissociation from estrogenic effects. *J Psychiatr Res*. 2009a;43:656-663.

McNamara RK, Able JA, Jandacek R, Rider T, Tso P, and Lindquist DM. Perinatal omega-3 fatty acid deficiency selectively reduces myo-inositol levels in the adult rat prefrontal cortex: An in vivo ^{1}H-MRS study. *J Lipid Res*. 2009b;50:405-411.

McNamara RK, Nandagopal JJ, Strakowski SM, and DelBello MP. Preventative strategies for early-onset bipolar disorder: towards a clinical staging model. *CNS Drugs*. 2010a;24:983-996.

McNamara RK, Jandacek R, Rider T, Tso P, Dwivedi Y, and Pandey GN. Selective deficits in erythrocyte docosahexaenoic acid composition in adult patients with bipolar disorder and major depressive disorder. *J Affect Disord*. 2010b;126:303-311.

McNamara RK, Rider T, Jandacek R, Tso P, Cole-Strauss A. and Lipton JW. Omega-3 fatty acid deficiency increases constitutive pro-inflammatory cytokine production in rats: Relationship with central serotonin turnover. *Prostaglandins Leukot Essent Fatty Acids*. 2010c;83:185-191.

McNamara RK, Able JA, Jandacek R, Rider T, Tso P, Eliassen J, Alfieri D, Weber W, Jarvis K, DelBello MP, Strakowski SM, and Adler CM. Docosahexaenoic acid supplementation increases prefrontal cortex activation during sustained attention in healthy boys: A placebo-controlled, dose-ranging, functional magnetic resonance imaging study. *Am J Clin Nutr*. 2010d;91:1060-1067.

McNamara RK and Jandacek R. Investigation of postmortem brain polyunsaturated fatty acid composition in psychiatric disorders: Limitations, challenges, and future directions. *J Psychiatry Res*. 2011;45:44-46.

McNamara RK, Able JA, Liu Y, Jandacek R, Rider T, Tso P, and Lipton JW. Omega-3 fatty acid deficiency does not alter the effects of chronic fluoxetine treatment on central serotonin turnover or behavior in the forced swim test in female rats. *Pharmacol Biochem Behav*. 2013a;114:1-8.

McNamara RK. Long-chain omega-3 fatty acid deficiency in mood disorders: Rationale for treatment and prevention. *Curr Drug Discov Technol.* 2013a;10:233-244.

McNamara RK. Deciphering the role of docosahexaenoic acid in brain maturation and pathology with magnetic resonance imaging. *Prostaglandins Leukot Essent Fatty Acids*. 2013b;88:33-42.

McNamara RK, Jandacek R, Rider T, Tso P, Weber W, Chu W-J, Strakowski SM, Adler CM, and DelBello MP. Low docosahexaenoic acid status is associated with reduced indices of cortical integrity in the anterior cingulate of healthy boys: A 1H MRS study. *Nutr Neurosci*. 2013;16:183-190.

McNamara RK, Strimpfel J, Jandacek R, Rider T, Tso P, Welge JA, Strawn JR, and DelBello MP. Detection and treatment of long-chain omega-3 fatty acid deficiency in adolescents with SSRI-resistant major depressive disorder. *PharmaNutrition*. 2014;2:38-46.

Mellor JE, Laugharne JD, and Peet M. Schizophrenic symptoms and dietary intake of *n*-3 fatty acids. *Schizoph. Res.* 1995;18:85-86.

Ment LR, Kesler S, Vohr B, Katz KH, Baumgartner H, Schneider KC, Delancy S, Silbereis J, Duncan CC, Constable RT, Makuch RW, and Reiss AL. Longitudinal brain volume changes in preterm and term control subjects during late childhood and adolescence. *Pediatrics*. 2009;123:503-511.

Meyers J, Classi P, Wietecha L, and Candrilli S. Economic burden and comorbidities of attention-deficit/hyperactivity disorder among pediatric patients hospitalized in the United States. *Child Adolesc Psychiatry Ment* Health. 2010;4:31.

Mirnikjoo B, Brown SE, Kim HF, Marangell LB, Sweatt JD, and Weeber EJ. Protein kinase inhibition by omega-3 fatty acids. *J Biol Chem.* 2001;276:10888-10896.

Moriguchi T, Greiner RS, and Salem N Jr. Behavioral deficits associated with dietary induction of decreased brain docosahexaenoic acid concentration. *J Neurochem*. 2000;75:2563-2573.

Moriguchi T and Salem N Jr. Recovery of brain docosahexaenoate leads to recovery of spatial task performance. *J Neurochem*. 2003;87:297-309.

Mullen KM, Vohr BR, Katz KH, Schneider KC, Lacadie C, Hampson M, Makuch RW, and Reiss AL, Constable RT, Ment LR. Preterm birth results in alterations in neural connectivity at age 16 years. *Neuroimage.* 2011;54:2563-2570.

Murakami K, Miyake Y, Sasaki S, Tanaka K, and Arakawa M. Fish and *n*-3 polyunsaturated fatty acid intake and depressive symptoms: Ryukyus Child Health Study. *Pediatrics.* 2010;126:623-630.

Nagy Z, Westerberg H, Skare S, Andersson JL, Lilja A, Flodmark O, Fernell E, Holmberg K, Bohm B, Forssberg H, Lagercrantz H, and Klingberg T. Preterm children have disturbances of white matter at 11 years of age as shown by diffusion tensor imaging. *Pediatr Res.* 2003;54:672-679.

Nemets H, Nemets B, Apter A, Bracha Z, and Belmaker RH. Omega-3 treatment of childhood depression: a controlled, double-blind pilot study. *Am J Psychiatry.* 2006;163:1098-1100.

Nestler EJ and Carlezon WA Jr. The mesolimbic dopamine reward circuit in depression. *Biol Psychiatry.* 2006;59:1151-1159.

Neuringer M, Connor WE, Lin DS, Barstad L, and Luck S. Biochemical and functional effects of prenatal and postnatal omega 3 fatty acid deficiency on retina and brain in rhesus monkeys. *Proc Natl Acad Sci U S A.* 1986;83:4021-4025.

Nishikawa M, Kimura S, and Akaike N. Facilitatory effect of docosahexaenoic acid on *N*-methyl-D-aspartate response in pyramidal neurones of rat cerebral cortex. *J Physiol.* 1994;475:83-93.

Noaghiul S and Hibbeln JR. Cross-national comparisons of seafood consumption and rates of bipolar disorders. *Am J Psychiatry.* 2003;160:2222-2227.

Nosarti C, Al-Asady MH, Frangou S, Stewart AL, Rifkin L, and Murray RM. Adolescents who were born very preterm have decreased brain volumes. *Brain.* 2002;125:1616-1623.

Nosarti C, Reichenberg A, Murray RM, Cnattingius S, Lambe MP, Yin L, MacCabe J, Rifkin L, and Hultman CM. Preterm birth and psychiatric disorders in young adult life. *Arch Gen Psychiatry.* 2012;69:E1-8.

Oddy WH, Hickling S, Smith MA, O'Sullivan TA, Robinson M, de Klerk NH, Beilin LJ, Mori TA, Syrette J, Zubrick SR, and Silburn SR. Dietary intake of omega-3 fatty acids and risk of depressive symptoms in adolescents. *Depress Anxiety.* 2011;28:582-588.

Olsen SF, Østerdal ML, Salvig JD, Weber T, Tabor A, and Secher NJ. Duration of pregnancy in relation to fish oil supplementation and habitual fish intake: a randomised clinical trial with fish oil. *Eur J Clin Nutr.* 2007;61:976-985.

Olsen SF, Sørensen JD, Secher NJ, Hedegaard M, Henriksen TB, Hansen HS, and Grant A. Randomised controlled trial of effect of fish-oil supplementation on pregnancy duration. *Lancet.* 1992;339(8800):1003-1007.

Orr SK, Palumbo S, Bosetti F, Mount HT, Kang JX, Greenwood CE, Ma DW, Serhan CN, and Bazinet RP. Unesterified docosahexaenoic acid is protective in neuroinflammation. *J Neurochem*. 2013;127:378-393.

Osby U, Brandt L, Correia N, Ekbom A, and Sparén P. Excess mortality in bipolar and unipolar disorder in Sweden. *Arch Gen Psychiatry*. 2001;58:844-850.

Otto SJ, van Houwelingen AC, Badart-Smook A, and Hornstra G. Changes in the maternal essential fatty acid profile during early pregnancy and the relation of the profile to diet. *Am J Clin Nutr*. 2001;73:302-307.

Ouellet M, Emond V, Chen CT, Julien C, Bourasset F, Oddo S, LaFerla F, Bazinet RP, and Calon F. Diffusion of docosahexaenoic and eicosapentaenoic acids through the blood-brain barrier: An in situ cerebral perfusion study. *Neurochem Int*. 2009;55:476-482.

Ozyurt B, Sarsilmaz M, Akpolat N, Ozyurt H, Akyol O, Herken H, and Kus I. The protective effects of omega-3 fatty acids against MK-801-induced neurotoxicity in prefrontal cortex of rat. *Neurochem Int.* 2007;50:196-202.

Paus T, Zijdenbos A, Worsley K, Collins DL, Blumenthal J, Giedd JN, Rapoport JL, and Evans AC. Structural maturation of neural pathways in children and adolescents: in vivo study. *Science.* 1999;283:1908-1911.

Peet M, Brind J, Ramchand CN, Shah S, and Vankar GK. Two double-blind placebo-controlled pilot studies of eicosapentaenoic acid in the treatment of schizophrenia. *Schizophr Res*. 2001;49:243-251.

Peet M. International variations in the outcome of schizophrenia and the prevalence of depression in relation to national dietary practices: an ecological analysis. Br *J Psychiatry* 2004;184:404-408.

Perlis RH, Dennehy EB, Miklowitz DJ, Delbello MP, Ostacher M, Calabrese JR, Ametrano RM, Wisniewski SR, Bowden CL, Thase ME, Nierenberg AA, and Sachs G. Retrospective age at onset of bipolar disorder and outcome during two-year follow-up: results from the STEP-BD study. *Bipolar Disord.* 2009;11:391-400.

Petanjek Z, Judaš M, Šimic G, Rasin MR, Uylings HB, Rakic P, and Kostovic I. Extraordinary neoteny of synaptic spines in the human prefrontal cortex. *Proc Natl Acad Sci U S A*. 2011;108(32):13281-13286.

Peterson BS, Vohr B, Staib LH, Cannistraci CJ, Dolberg A, Schneider KC, Katz KH, Westerveld M, Sparrow S, Anderson AW, Duncan CC, Makuch

RW, Gore JC, and Ment LR. Regional brain volume abnormalities and long-term cognitive outcome in preterm infants. *JAMA*. 2000;284:1939-1947.

Pifferi F, Roux F, Langelier B, Alessandri JM, Vancassel S, Jouin M, Lavialle M, and Guesnet P. (*n*-3) polyunsaturated fatty acid deficiency reduces the expression of both isoforms of the brain glucose transporter GLUT1 in rats. *J Nutr*. 2005;135:2241-2246.

Polanczyk G, de Lima MS, Horta BL, Biederman J, and Rohde LA. The worldwide prevalence of ADHD: a systematic review and metaregression analysis. *Am J Psychiatry*. 2007;164:942-948.

Pottala JV, Talley JA, Churchill SW, Lynch DA, von Schacky C, and Harris WS. Red blood cell fatty acids are associated with depression in a case-control study of adolescents. *Prostaglandins Leukot Essent Fatty Acids*. 2012;86:161-165.

Putnam JC, Carlson SE, DeVoe PW, and Barness LA. The effect of variations in dietary fatty acids on the fatty acid composition of erythrocyte phosphatidylcholine and phosphatidylethanolamine in human infants. *Am J Clin Nutr*. 1982;36:106-114.

Raeder MB, Steen VM, Vollset SE, and Bjelland I. Associations between cod liver oil use and symptoms of depression: the Hordaland Health Study. *J Affect Disord* 2007;101:245-249.

Ranjekar PK, Hinge A, Hegde MV, Ghate M, Kale A, Sitasawad S, Wagh UV, Debsikdar VB, and Mahadik SP. Decreased antioxidant enzymes and membrane essential polyunsaturated fatty acids in schizophrenic and bipolar mood disorder patients. *Psychiatry Res*. 2003;121:109-122.

Rao JS, Ertley RN, DeMar JC Jr, Rapoport SI, Bazinet RP, and Lee HJ. Dietary *n*-3 PUFA deprivation alters expression of enzymes of the arachidonic and docosahexaenoic acid cascades in rat frontal cortex. *Mol. Psychiatry*. 2007a;12:151-157.

Rao JS, Ertley RN, Lee HJ, DeMar JC Jr, Arnold JT, Rapoport SI, and Bazinet RP. *n*-3 polyunsaturated fatty acid deprivation in rats decreases frontal cortex BDNF via a p38 MAPK-dependent mechanism. *Mol Psychiatry*. 2007b;12:36-46.

Rapoport SI, Chang MC, and Spector AA. Delivery and turnover of plasma-derived essential PUFAs in mammalian brain. *J. Lipid Res*. 2001;42:678-685.

Rapoport SI, Ramadan E, and Basselin M. Docosahexaenoic acid (DHA) incorporation into the brain from plasma, as an in vivo biomarker of brain

DHA metabolism and neurotransmission. *Prostaglandins Other Lipid Mediat.* 2011;96:109-113.

Reddy RD, Keshavan MS, and Yao JK. Reduced red blood cell membrane essential polyunsaturated fatty acids in first episode schizophrenia at neuroleptic-naive baseline. *Schizophr Bull.* 2004;30:901-911.

Reisbick S, Neuringer M, Gohl E, Wald R, and Anderson GJ. Visual attention in infant monkeys: effects of dietary fatty acids and age. *Dev Psychol.* 1997;33:387-395.

Reisbick S, Neuringer M, Hasnain R, and Connor WE. Home cage behavior of rhesus monkeys with long-term deficiency of omega-3 fatty acids. *Physiol Behav.* 1994;55:231-239.

Reisbick S, Neuringer M, Hasnain R, and Connor WE. Polydipsia in rhesus monkeys deficient in omega-3 fatty acids. *Physiol Behav.* 1990;47:315-323.

Richardson AJ, Burton JR, Sewell RP, Spreckelsen TF, and Montgomery P. Docosahexaenoic acid for reading, cognition and behavior in children aged 7-9 years: a randomized, controlled trial (the DOLAB Study). *PLoS One.* 2012;7:e43909.

Rosa Neto P, Lou H, Cumming P, Pryds O, and Gjedde A. Methylphenidate-evoked potentiation of extracellular dopamine in the brain of adolescents with premature birth: correlation with attentional deficit. *Ann.N. Y. Acad. Sci.* 2002;965:434-439.

Ryan AS, Astwood JD, Gautier S, Kuratko CN, Nelson EB, and Salem N Jr. Effects of long-chain polyunsaturated fatty acid supplementation on neurodevelopment in childhood: a review of human studies. *Prostaglandins Leukot Essent Fatty Acids.* 2010;82:305-314.

Rzehak P, Heinrich J, Klopp N, Schaeffer L, Hoff S, Wolfram G, Illig T, and Linseisen J. Evidence for an association between genetic variants of the fatty acid desaturase 1 fatty acid desaturase 2 (FADS1 FADS2) gene cluster and the fatty acid composition of erythrocyte membranes. *Br J Nutr.* 2009;101:20-26.

Sacher J, Neumann J, Fünfstück T, Soliman A, Villringer A, and Schroeter ML. Mapping the depressed brain: a meta-analysis of structural and functional alterations in major depressive disorder. *J Affect Disord.* 2012;140:142-148.

Sakamoto T, Cansev M, and Wurtman RJ. Oral supplementation with docosahexaenoic acid and uridine-5'-monophosphate increases dendritic spine density in adult gerbil hippocampus. *Brain Res.* 2007;1182:50-59.

Salvig JD and Lamont RF. Evidence regarding an effect of marine *n*-3 fatty acids on preterm birth: a systematic review and meta-analysis. *Acta Obstet Gynecol* Scand. 2011;90:825-838.

Samieri C, Maillard P, Crivello F, Proust-Lima C, Peuchant E, Helmer C, Amieva H, Allard M, Dartigues JF, Cunnane SC, Mazoyer BM, and Barberger-Gateau P. Plasma long-chain omega-3 fatty acids and atrophy of the medial temporal lobe. Neurology. 2012;79:642-650.

Sands SA, Reid KJ, Windsor SL, and Harris WS. The impact of age, body mass index, and fish intake on the EPA and DHA content of human erythrocytes. *Lipids.* 2005;40:343-347.

Sarkadi-Nagy E, Wijendran V, Diau GY, Chao AC, Hsieh AT, Turpeinen A, Lawrence P, Nathanielsz PW, and Brenna JT. Formula feeding potentiates docosahexaenoic and arachidonic acid biosynthesis in term and preterm baboon neonates. *J Lipid Res.* 2004;45:71-80.

Sarkadi-Nagy E, Wijendran V, Diau GY, Chao AC, Hsieh AT, Turpeinen A, Nathanielsz PW, and Brenna JT. The influence of prematurity and long chain polyunsaturate supplementation in 4-week adjusted age baboon neonate brain and related tissues. *Pediatr Res.* 2003;54:244-252.

Sarris J, Mischoulon D, and Schweitzer I. Omega-3 for bipolar disorder: meta-analyses of use in mania and bipolar depression. *J Clin Psychiatry.* 2012;73:81-86.

Schafer RJ, Lacadie C, Vohr B, Kesler SR, Katz KH, Schneider KC, Pugh KR, Makuch RW, Reiss AL, Constable RT, and Ment LR. Alterations in functional connectivity for language in prematurely born adolescents. *Brain.* 2009;132:661-670.

Scholtz SA, Colombo J, and Carlson SE. Clinical overview of effects of dietary long-chain polyunsaturated fatty acids during the perinatal period. *Nestle Nutr* Inst Workshop Ser. 2013;77:145-154.

Sichert-Hellert W, Wicher M, and Kersting M. Age and time trends in fish consumption pattern of children and adolescents, and consequences for the intake of long-chain *n*-3 polyunsaturated fatty acids. *Eur J Clin Nutr.* 2009;63:1071-1075.

Silk TJ, Vance A, Rinehart N, Bradshaw JL, and Cunnington R. White-matter abnormalities in attention deficit hyperactivity disorder: a diffusion tensor imaging study. *Hum Brain Mapp.* 2009;30:2757-2765.

Smithers LG, Gibson RA, and Makrides M. Maternal supplementation with docosahexaenoic acid during pregnancy does not affect early visual development in the infant: a randomized controlled trial. *Am J Clin Nutr.* 2011;93:1293-1299.

Smyser CD, Snyder AZ, Shimony JS, Blazey TM, Inder TE, and Neil JJ. Effects of white matter injury on resting state fMRI measures in prematurely born infants. *PLoS One.* 2013;8:e68098.

Sowell ER, Thompson PM, Holmes CJ, Batth R, Jernigan TL, and Toga AW. Localizing age-related changes in brain structure between childhood and adolescence using statistical parametric mapping. *Neuroimage.* 1999;9:587-597.

Stein DJ. Depression, anhedonia, and psychomotor symptoms: the role of dopaminergic neurocircuitry. *CNS Spectr.* 2008;13:561-565.

Stewart AL, Rifkin L, Amess PN, Kirkbride V, Townsend JP, Miller DH, Lewis SW, Kingsley DP, Moseley IF, Foster O, and Murray RM. Brain structure and neurocognitive and behavioural function in adolescents who were born very preterm. *Lancet.* 1999;353:1653-1657.

Strakowski SM, Adler CM, Almeida J, Altshuler LL, Blumberg HP, Chang KD, DelBello MP, Frangou S, McIntosh A, Phillips ML, Sussman JE, and Townsend JD. The functional neuroanatomy of bipolar disorder: a consensus model. *Bipolar Disord.* 2012;14:313-325.

Su HM, Bernardo L, Mirmiran M, Ma XH, Corso TN, Nathanielsz PW, and Brenna JT. Bioequivalence of dietary alpha-linolenic and docosahexaenoic acids as sources of docosahexaenoate accretion in brain and associated organs of neonatal baboons. *Pediatr Res.* 1999;45:87-93.

Su KP, Huang SY, Peng CY, Lai HC, Huang CL, Chen YC, Aitchison KJ, and Pariante CM. Phospholipase A2 and cyclooxygenase 2 genes influence the risk of interferon-alpha-induced depression by regulating polyunsaturated fatty acids levels. *Biol Psychiatry.* 2010;67:550-557.

Sublette ME, Hibbeln JR, Galfalvy H, Oquendo MA, and Mann JJ. Omega-3 polyunsaturated essential fatty acid status as a predictor of future suicide risk. *Am J Psychiatry.* 2006;163:1100-1102.

Sullivan PF, Neale MC, and Kendler KS. Genetic epidemiology of major depression: review and meta-analysis. *Am. J. Psychiatry.* 2000;157:1552-1562.

Sun L, Cao Q, Long X, Sui M, Cao X, Zhu C, Zuo X, An L, Song Y, Zang Y, and Wang Y. Abnormal functional connectivity between the anterior cingulate and the default mode network in drug-naïve boys with attention deficit hyperactivity disorder. *Psychiatry Res.* 2012;201:120-127.

Suzuki H, Manabe S, Wada O, and Crawford MA. Rapid incorporation of docosahexaenoic acid from dietary sources into brain microsomal, synaptosomal and mitochondrial membranes in adult mice. *Int. J. Vitam. Nutr. Res.* 1997;67:272-278.

Swenne I, Rosling A, Tengblad S, and Vessby B. Omega-3 polyunsaturated essential fatty acids are associated with depression in adolescents with eating disorders and weight loss. *Acta Paediatr*. 2011;100:1610-1615.

Tanskanen A, Hibbeln JR, Tuomilehto J, Uutela A, Haukkala A, Viinamäki H, Lehtonen J, and Vartiainen E. Fish consumption and depressive symptoms in the general population in Finland. *Psychiatr Serv* 2001;52:529-531.

Tatebayashi Y, Nihonmatsu-Kikuchi N, Hayashi Y, Yu X, Soma M, and Ikeda K. Abnormal fatty acid composition in the frontopolar cortex of patients with affective disorders. *Transl Psychiatry*. 2013;2:e204.

Tian L, Jiang T, Wang Y, Zang Y, He Y, Liang M, Sui M, Cao Q, Hu S, Peng M, and Zhuo Y. Altered resting-state functional connectivity patterns of anterior cingulate cortex in adolescents with attention deficit hyperactivity disorder. *Neurosci Lett*. 2006;400:39-43.

Timonen M, Horrobin D, Jokelainen J, Laitinen J, Herva A, and Räsänen P. Fish consumption and depression: the Northern Finland 1966 birth cohort study. *J Affect Disord* 2004;82:447-452.

Tisserand DJ, Pruessner JC, Sanz Arigita EJ, van Boxtel MP, Evans AC, Jolles J, and Uylings HB. Regional frontal cortical volumes decrease differentially in aging: an MRI study to compare volumetric approaches and voxel-based morphometry. *Neuroimage*. 2002;17:657-669.

Titova OE, Sjögren P, Brooks SJ, Kullberg J, Ax E, Kilander L, Riserus U, Cederholm T, Larsson EM, Johansson L, Ahlström H, Lind L, Schiöth HB, and Benedict C. Dietary intake of eicosapentaenoic and docosahexaenoic acids is linked to gray matter volume and cognitive function in elderly. *Age* (Dordr). 2013;35:1495-1505.

Tsuang M. Schizophrenia: genes and environment. *Biol Psychiatry*. 2000;47:210-220.

Tsukada H, Kakiuchi T, Fukumoto D, Nishiyama S, and Koga K. Docosahexaenoic acid (DHA) improves the age-related impairment of the coupling mechanism between neuronal activation and functional cerebral blood flow response: a PET study in conscious monkeys. *Brain Res*. 2000;862:180-186.

Tuzun F, Kumral A, Dilek M, Ozbal S, Ergur B, Yesilirmak DC, Duman N, Yilmaz O, and Ozkan H. Maternal omega-3 fatty acid supplementation protects against lipopolysaccharide-induced white matter injury in the neonatal rat brain. *J Matern Fetal Neonatal Med*. 2012;25:849-854.

Ulmann L, Mimouni V, Roux S, Porsolt R, and Poisson JP. Brain and hippocampus fatty acid composition in phospholipid classes of aged-relative cognitive deficit rats. *Prostaglandins Leukot Essent Fatty Acids*. 2001;64:189-195.

Vaisman N, Kaysar N, Zaruk-Adasha Y, Pelled D, Brichon G, Zwingelstein G, and Bodennec J. Correlation between changes in blood fatty acid composition and visual sustained attention performance in children with inattention: effect of dietary *n*-3 fatty acids containing phospholipids. *Am J Clin Nutr*. 2008;87:1170-1180.

Vancassel S, Leman S, Hanonick L, Denis S, Roger J, Nollet M, Bodard S, Kousignian I, Belzung C, and Chalon S. *n*-3 polyunsaturated fatty acid supplementation reverses stress-induced modifications on brain monoamine levels in mice. *J Lipid Res*. 2008;49:340-348.

Vaswani M, Linda FK, and Ramesh S. Role of selective serotonin reuptake inhibitors in psychiatric disorders: a comprehensive review. *Prog Neuropsychopharmacol Biol Psychiatry*. 2003;27:85-102.

Virtanen JK, Siscovick DS, Lemaitre RN, Longstreth WT, Spiegelman D, Rimm EB, King IB, and Mozaffarian D. Circulating omega-3 polyunsaturated fatty acids and subclinical brain abnormalities on MRI in older adults: the Cardiovascular Health Study. *J Am Heart Assoc*. 2013;2:e000305.

Vita A, De Peri L, Deste G, and Sacchetti E. Progressive loss of cortical gray matter in schizophrenia: a meta-analysis and meta-regression of longitudinal MRI studies. *Transl Psychiatry*. 2013.

Walhovd KB, Storsve AB, Westlye LT, Drevon CA, and Fjell AM. Blood markers of fatty acids and vitamin D, cardiovascular measures, body mass index, and physical activity relate to longitudinal cortical thinning in normal aging. *Neurobiol Aging*. 2014;35:1055-1064.

White TP, Symington I, Castellanos NP, Brittain PJ, Froudist Walsh S, Nam KW, Sato JR, Allin MP, Shergill SS, Murray RM, Williams SC, and Nosarti C. Dysconnectivity of neurocognitive networks at rest in very-preterm born adults. *Neuroimage Clin*. 2014;4:352-365.

Williams C, Birch EE, Emmett PM, Northstone K, and Avon Longitudinal Study of Pregnancy and Childhood Study Team. Stereoacuity at age 3.5 y in children born full-term is associated with prenatal and postnatal dietary factors: a report from a population-based cohort study. *Am J Clin Nutr*. 2001;73:316-322.

Wozniak J, Biederman J, Mick E, Waxmonsky J, Hantsoo L, Best C, Cluette-Brown JE, and Laposata M. Omega-3 fatty acid monotherapy for pediatric bipolar disorder: a prospective open-label trial. *Eur Neuropsychopharmacol*. 2007;17:440-447.

Wu A, Ying Z and Gomez-Pinilla F. Dietary omega-3 fatty acids normalize BDNF levels, reduce oxidative damage, and counteract learning disability after traumatic brain injury in rats. *J Neurotrauma*. 2004;21:1457-1467.

Wu EQ, Birnbaum HG, Shi L, Ball DE, Kessler RC, Moulis M, and Aggarwal J. The economic burden of schizophrenia in the United States in 2002. *J Clin Psychiatry*. 2005;66:1122-1129.

Ximenes da Silva A, Lavialle F, Gendrot G, Guesnet P, Alessandri JM, and Lavialle M. Glucose transport and utilization are altered in the brain of rats deficient in *n*-3 polyunsaturated fatty acids. *J Neurochem*. 2002;81:1328-1337.

Yao JK, Leonard S, Reddy RD. Membrane phospholipid abnormalities in postmortem brains from schizophrenic patients. *Schizophr Res*. 2000;42:7-17.

Yavin E, Brand A, and Green P. Docosahexaenoic acid abundance in the brain: a biodevice to combat oxidative stress. *Nutr Neurosci*. 2002;5:149-157.

Yavin E, Himovichi E, and Eilam R. Delayed cell migration in the developing rat brain following maternal omega 3 alpha linolenic acid dietary deficiency. *Neuroscience*. 2009;162:1011-1122.

Yoshida S, Yasuda A, Kawazato H, Sakai K, Shimada T, Takeshita M, Yuasa S, Kobayashi T, Watanabe S, and Okuyama H. Synaptic vesicle ultrastructural changes in the rat hippocampus induced by a combination of alpha-linolenate deficiency and a learning task. *J Neurochem*. 1997;68:1261-1268.

Zimmer L, Delion-Vancassel S, Durand G, Guilloteau D, Bodard S, Besnard JC, and Chalon S. Modification of dopamine neurotransmission in the nucleus accumbens of rats deficient in *n*-3 polyunsaturated fatty acids. *J Lipid Res*. 2000b;41:32-40.

Zimmer L, Delpal S, Guilloteau D, Aioun J, Durand G, and Chalon S. Chronic *n*-3 polyunsaturated fatty acid deficiency alters dopamine vesicle density in the rat frontal cortex. *Neurosci Lett*. 2000a;284:25-28.

Zimmer L, Hembert S, Durand G, Breton P, Guilloteau D, Besnard JC, and Chalon S. Chronic *n*-3 polyunsaturated fatty acid diet-deficiency acts on dopamine metabolism in the rat frontal cortex: a microdialysis study. *Neurosci Lett*. 1998;240:177-181.

Zimmer L, Vancassel S, Cantagrel S, Breton P, Delamanche S, Guilloteau D, Durand G, and Chalon S. The dopamine mesocorticolimbic pathway is affected by deficiency in *n*-3 polyunsaturated fatty acids. *Am J Clin Nutr*. 2002;75:662-667.

Zugno AI, Chipindo HL, Volpato AM, Budni J, Steckert AV, de Oliveira MB, Heylmann AS, da Rosa Silveira F, Mastella GA, Maravai SG, Wessler PG, Binatti AR, Panizzutti B, Schuck PF, Quevedo J, and Gama CS. Omega-3 prevents behavior response and brain oxidative damage in the ketamine model of schizophrenia. *Neuroscience.* 2014;259:223-231.

In: Research Trends in Behavior … ISBN: 978-1-63485-461-0
Editor: Miao-Kun Sun

Chapter 3

EXECUTIVE FUNCTIONS AND THEIR ASSESSMENT IN CHILDREN AND ADOLESCENTS

Trinidad García, Celestino Rodríguez*, Paloma González-Castro and Débora Areces
University of Oviedo, Spain

ABSTRACT

Executive functions involve a series of cognitive, behavioral and affective-emotional components, which play an important role regulating and organizing one´s behavior in a wide range of situations, especially in those that require a creative and novel approach. The impact of these components is especially noticeable either on social, academic and clinical settings. This has led many authors to consider executive functions as a core aspect predicting social adaptation, as well as an important asset in the diagnosis and intervention in several childhood and adolescence disorders. This prominence given to executive functions suggests the need for reliable and valid assessment tools, and even more importantly, the need for an adequate body of information that helps researchers and professionals to successfully interpret results from

* Correspondence and requests for reprints: Celestino Rodríguez PhD. Address: Faculty of Psychology, University of Oviedo, Plaza Feijoo s/n, 33003 Oviedo (Asturias), Spain. Ph: +34985103411; Fax: +34 985 10 41 40. E-mail address: rodriguezcelestino@uniovi.es

empiric evidence. This chapter is aimed at addressing both aspects. Thus, we focus on analyzing the main features of the assessment tools available today and to what extent they are suitable for their application in clinical and educational settings, paying special attention to new perspectives and instruments. Finally, we outline some suggestions intended to improve election, application and interpretation of the results gathered in the evaluation process.

Keywords: assessment, behavior, executive functions, performance, validity

1. Introduction

Executive functions are responsible for the generation, supervision, regulation, performance, and readjustment of behavior to achieve a goal, especially in situations requiring a novel and creative approach (Verdejo-García and Bechara, 2010). In this sense, a wide range of aspects such as goal setting, hypothesis formulation, planning, attention, monitoring, problem solving, cognitive flexibility, working memory, response inhibition, or emotional control are intimately linked to this concept (Korzeniowski, 2011). These components have been demonstrated to play an important role in learning processes, mainly in areas such as calculus and mathematical problem-solving or reading-writing at early ages (Lee et al., 2009; Mizuno et al., 2011; Tolletal, 2012; Van der Ven, et al., 2013), as well as in the differential diagnosis of numerous neurodevelopmental disorders, such as Autism Spectrum Disorders (Geurts and Marlies, 2012; Robinson et al., 2009), mental retardation (Danielsson et al., 2012) or ADHD (García et al., 2013, 2014; Hale et al., 2011; Shimoni, Engel-Yeger and Tirosh, 2012).

This has led many authors to designate executive functions as superordinal processes. This affirmation has been supported by several neuroanatomical studies, which showed the relevance of the prefrontal area and its connections as the neurological basis for executive control components (Lozano and Ostrosky, 2011; Stuss and Knight, 2013; Wolosin et al., 2009). These studies also confirmed that executive functioning is a non-unitary entity, but made up of diverse components. It is precisely the complexity of this construct which makes necessary its subdivision into assessable units in order to facilitate its study and analyze its relationship with the observed behavior.

There have been numerous attempts to classify the executive functions, often with mixed results. Some of the classification systems proposed were based on functional criteria, like the differentiation between "hot" and "cool" functions (Brock et al., 2009; Chan et al., 2007; Dolcos and McCarthy, 2006; Tirapú-Ustárroz et al., 2008), or between strategic or dynamic functions (Huettel et al., 2004), whereas others have emphasized their neuroanatomical correlates (Slachevsky et al., 2005). These studies have confirmed the existence of different components within the executive functions, as they are of a cognitive, behavioral, and emotional nature. Working memory, organization and planning, response inhibition, cognitive flexibility, and attention capacity have been the most extensively studied functions, which most of the assessment tools have been developed for (Diamond, 2013; Korzeniowski, 2011; Toplak et al., 2009; Van der Sluis et al., 2007; Van De Voorde et al., 2010).

2. Assessment of Executive functions: Traditional Measures

Although different criteria have been used to classify the assessment measures of executive functions, the classification provided in this chapter is based on the distinction between performance-based instruments (also called neuropsychological measures) and measures based on behavior observation, commonly referred to as questionnaires. Once we identify and describe briefly the most widely known assessment tools, we focus on the analysis of the correspondence between different types of measures as a core aspect in the current scientific scene.

3. Neuropsychological Measures

These are individual tests or batteries made up of different tasks that provide a series of objective indicators related to individuals' performance, generally response times, number of errors, and omissions. We present the most frequently employed tests in recent years and describe a relatively new tool, based on Instrumental Activities of Daily Life (IADL).

Individual tests have been designed to assess particular components of executive functions. Examples of this sort of measures are the Stroop Color and Word Test (Stroop, 1935; Golden, 1974; Martín et al., 2012), the Matching Familiar Figures Test (MFFT; Kagan, 1965) and the 20-kern

Matching Familiar Figures Test (MFF-20; Cairos and Cammock, 1982; 2002), the Simon Task (Simon, 1969; Simon and Berbaum, 1990), or the Stop Task (Logan et al., 1984; Schachar et al., 2000) to assess response inhibition; Continuous Performance Test (CPT) such as the TOVA test (Test of Variables of Attention; Greenberg, 1996), the Conners Continuous Performance Test 2nd Edition (Conners CPT-II; Conners, 2004) or the AULA Nesplora [Nesplora Classroom] (Climent and Bánterla, 2011) to evaluate inhibition and attention; the Working Memory Test Battery for Children (WMTB-C: Pickering and Gathercole, 2001), or Digit Span subtests, such as the Automated Working Memory Assessment test (AWMA: Alloway, 2007) and WISC-IV Working Memory Index (Wechsler, 2003), or the Keep Track test (Van der Sluis et al., 2007) to assess working memory; the Tower of Hanoi (ToH: Borys et al., 1892) and Tower of London (ToL: Shallice, 1982) to evaluate planning; or the Wisconsin Card Sorting Test (WCST: Grant and Berg, 1948; Heaton, 1981), the Trail Making Test (TMT: Reitan, 1958; Barncord, 2002), the Comprehensive Trail-making Test (CTMT: Reynolds, 2002) and the Children Coloured Trail Test (CCTT: Llorente, Williams, Satz, and D`Elia, 2003), or the Symbol Shifting (Van der Sluis et al., 2007) and Animal Shifting (Toll et al., 2011) to obtain a measure of cognitive flexibility.

Performance batteries commonly incorporate some of the previous individual measures. These instruments allow a global assessment of the executive functions in children and adolescents. The most extensively studied batteries are the Delis-Kaplan Executive Function System (D-KEFS: Delis et al., 2001), the Cambridge Neuropsychological Automated Battery-CANTAB (Strauss, Sherman and Spreen, 2006), or the Behavioral Assessment of the Dysexecutive Syndrome for Children (BADS-C; Kobayashi and Kobayashi, 2007).

These tests have been broadly used, mainly in clinical practice, to appraise the presence of executive deficits, and have generally been shown to be useful to detect deficits in executive functioning. However, they have been criticized because of their low "ecological validity" (Chevignard et al., 2010; Gioia et al., 2010; Lee, 2011; Lezak et al., 2012). This term refers to the property of a test to establish a functional relationship between a person's performance on the test and the person's behavioral expression in relevant life settings, such as social relationships or academic performance (Burin et al., 2007). Results from previous studies found a low association between both aspects. The origin of the tests (some of them have been designed to assess constructs different from executive functions, mainly intelligence), the multitude of capacities associated with executive functions, the involvement of other cognitive, verbal, perceptive, or motor aspects in the performance of these tasks, the possible effect of practice, the quantitative nature and the high degree of structure that commonly characterizes evaluation situations, are some of the reasons argued to attribute a low ecological validity to these measures.

3.1. Performance Tasks Based on Instrumental Activities of Daily Life (IADL): An Attempt to Reach Ecological Validity

In response to the criticized ecological validity of the above-mentioned tests, in the past decades, a new type of measures emerged, based on the performance of daily life tasks. These tasks, also performance-based, imply the accomplishment of daily tasks, attempting to reproduce similar conditions to those occurring in real settings. Based on the instrumental activities of daily life, (IALDS), these tests allow one to identify the strengths and weaknesses of the participants being assessed in various domains of executive functions, examining the factors that favor or hinder their performance.

The most well known measures in the assessment of children and adolescents are the Assessment of Motor and Processing Skills- AMPS (Fingerhut, Madill, Darrah, Hodge, and Warren, 2002) and the Children´s Kitchen Task Assessment- CKTA (Rocke et al., 2008). CKTA is the most widely used test, and assesses the level of help and supervision that children and adolescents need to perform a cooking task, estimated by the number of clues they need to complete the task. This provides an estimation of the cognitive and executive aspects present in effective task performance. These tests frequently include the components of initiation, planning/seriation, judgment/confidence, organization, and completion.

In spite of certain advance of this type of instruments in terms of ecological validity, it is a fact that this kind of measures has not been widely applied. As they also involve an excessive structure, and include a very reduced range of instrumental activities of daily life, or activities that are not very common in our context at these ages (such as the cooking task), they are not a true alternative to traditional performance measures.

4. Measures Based on Observation

As the practice of executive functions is not only reflected in cognitive aspects, but also in social and emotional aspects—such as accepting other people's viewpoint or proposing alternatives to solve a problem, regulating one's emotional expressions or behavior, remembering certain rules or directives, inhibiting impulses, adapting to new settings or flexibly shifting one's behavior in changing situations—an exhaustive assessment of the executive functions should take these aspects into account. In this sense, an alternative to performance-based measures is to use behavior-rating scales, which allow one to determine the extent to which the behaviors displayed by children and adolescents at home and at school are indicative of deficits related to executive functions.

This kind of measures has been developed extensively in recent years (Egeland and Fallmyr, 2010; Huizinga and Smidts, 2011; Mares et al., 2007). Their goal is to assess the executive functions by means of behavior observation in real settings, mainly by means of information provided by families and teaching staff about the presence of certain problem behaviors related to the executive functions. The most well-known standardized assessment tools are: the Child Behavior Checklist (CBCL; Achenbach, 1991), the Children´s Executive Functions Scale (CEFS; Silver et al., 1993), the Behavior Rating Inventory of Executive Functions (BRIEF; Gioia et al., 2000), the Child Behavior Questionnaire (CBQ; Rothbart et al., 2001), the Behavioral Assessment of the Dysexecutive Syndrome for Children (BADSC: Emslie et al., 2003), the Children Executive Function Inventory (CHEXI; Thorell and Nyberg, 2008), and the Barkley Deficits in Executive Functioning Scale - Children and Adolescents (BDEFS-CA: Barkley, 2012).

5. Correspondence between both Types of Measures

Although the use of the behavior rating scales mentioned above is widely spread, concern about executive functions assessment is still a recurring issue. Among the main reasons for this concern is the low correspondence found between children's and adolescents' performance in these tasks and the difficulties observed in diverse daily life settings (Gioia et al., 2010; Lezak et al., 2012), as well as the low agreement found in some cases between the information provided by different informants -mainly families and teaching staff- (Bishop, 2011; McAuley et al., 2010; Salbach-Andrae et al., 2009; Toplak et al., 2009). On the one hand, some studies have reported significant, but low to moderate associations between the data gathered by means of neuropsychological tasks and observation-based measures. Authors like Lezak et al., (2012) suggest, however, that this low correspondence between measures may be due to the conditions in which the performance tests are administered, characterized by being highly structured situations of face-to-face interaction with minimum levels of distraction. These settings differ considerably from most of the daily settings in which the children and adolescents are immersed, like home, school and social environments. On the other hand, it has been proposed that the low agreement found between different informants in the observation scales could be related to the fact that both daily life settings (school and home) differ in terms of the informational spaces implied, and this leads to different processing demands. In this sense, the demand for executive activity would be heterogeneous in both spaces, depending on factors such as their novelty, or the structured, threatening, or cognitive demanding that these spaces are perceived by children and adolescents (Ardila, 2008; Chan et al., 2007).

6. New Perspectives in the Assessment of Executive Functions: AULA Nesplora

In view of the aforementioned limitations, other assessment techniques and sources of information should be taken into account, especially considering that neuropsychological measures do not always predict the daily behavior of children and adolescents.

AULA Nesplora system (Climent and Bánterla, 2011) has been a step forward towards the achievement of greater ecological validity in neuropsychological measures. It allows us to assess problems of attention and inhibition in children in an environment of virtual reality, replicating as closely as possible the conditions of a classroom (see Figure 1). It includes special glasses with movement sensors and headphones. While the child performs the test, a series of visual and auditory distracters, similar to those that might be found in a real classroom, are presented at different time intervals (i.e., in Figure 1 a classmate stands up and has a walk around the class). Therefore, the child faces the task under very similar conditions to those faced in daily life. This system is especially useful to assess visual, auditory, and mixed attention, tendency to distraction, excessive motor activity, and processing speed in a test lasting less than 20 minutes. AULA has been validated in a sample of

1500 students from 6 to 16 years in Spain. It has a sensitivity of .95 and a specificity of .91, showing a high convergent validity with Conners´CPT (Diaz-Orueta et al., 2012; Diaz-Orueta et al., 2014; Iriarte et al., 2012).

The results are clearly displayed in graphs and contain explanatory text for each variable, which makes it easier to interpret the results of the evaluation. This tool has been used in the diagnosis of ADHD, where it differentiated between ADHD children with and without pharmacological treatment for a wide range of measures related to inattention, impulsivity, processing speed, motor activity, and quality of attention focus (Díaz-Orueta et al., 2012, 2014). Moreover, the AULA showed differences by gender and correlation to Perceptual Reasoning and Working Memory indexes of the WISC-IV, supporting the relevance of IQ measures in the understanding of cognitive performance in ADHD. In this last study, advantages of the AULA versus Conners' CPT are also discussed in terms of ecological validity and specificity.

On the basis of these findings, it would seem that neuropsychological evaluation continues being an important part of the protocol to the understanding and appropriate identification of executive functions deficits, but lack of ecological validity of ordinary psycho-educational batteries has opened the door to other types of tools, such as computerized and Virtual Reality tests.

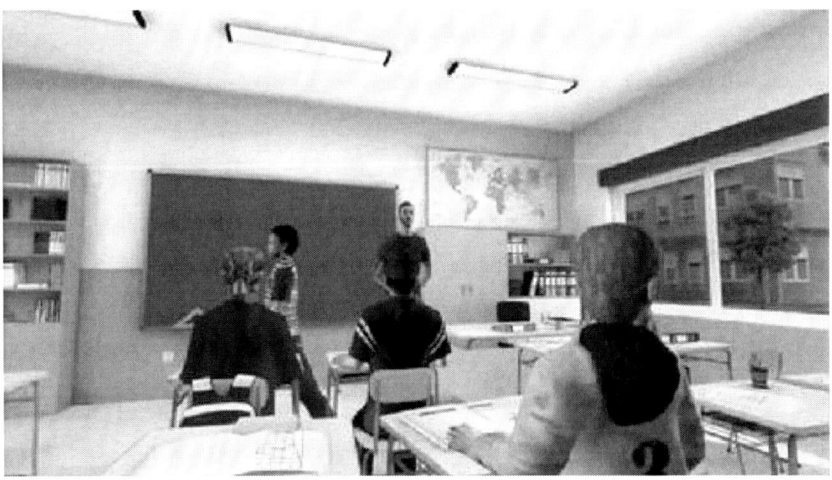

Figure 1. General view of AULA from the perspective of the child.

CONCLUSION

In view of the well-known relevance of the different components of executive functions as determining factors of behavior in childhood and adolescence, this chapter aimed at describing and analyzing the main features of the most widely spread assessment tools used to evaluate this construct in childhood and adolescence. Placing especial emphasis on the possible difficulties that arises from the use of these methods and techniques, we reached the following conclusions: firstly, in addition to the detection of possible executive deficits based on performance, it is essential to identify the impact of these problems on the functional aspects of daily life (Huizinga and Smidts, 2011; Egeland and Fallmyr, 2010). Measures based on the observation (behavior rating scales), suppose an alternative to neuropsychological tests. Nevertheless, the low correspondence between performance-based measures and behavior observation is one of the most important barriers to overcome today. Establish an adequate correspondence between the information provided by both types of measures is one of the main challenges in this sense; and second, in spite of the fact that numerous assessment tools are available today, the need for a more ecological orientation in the assessment of executive functions leads the way to new trends in evaluation, as the aforementioned AULA Nesplora (Climent and Bánterla, 2012).

However, authors such as García-Molina, Tirapu-Ustárroz and Roig-Rovira (2007) note that the ecological validity in the assessment of executive functions does not depend exclusively on the measures administered, but on an adequate contextualization of the information gathered. These authors point out that aspects such as the context of the assessment (i.e., very different protocols are required for clinical and educational assessment), the goal of the assessment (i.e., to establish a profile of the different executive components or to predict a daily functioning), or the target population, must be considered in order to achieve a complete evaluation. Being knowledgeable of the reality in which the subject is immersed, along with his or her personality characteristics, is also essential for a better understanding of the findings of the evaluation.

Taking into account these aspects, the recommendations derived from the scientific evidence imply exploring the entire range of executive components through representative indexes, paying a special attention to the cognitive, behavioral, and affective correlates of the construct, combining information from diverse assessment techniques, contexts and informants. Likewise, it is necessary to continue to advance in the design of more ecologically valid assessment tools, as well deepen in the study of executive functions, their characteristics and behavioral expressions in order to achieve a theoretical framework as comprehensive as possible. Only a solid framework on executive functions will allow researchers and professionals in different spheres to orient evaluation process and interpret the results in an appropriate way.

REFERENCES

Achenbach, T. M. (1991). Integrative guide for the 1991 CBCL/4-18, YSR and TRF profiles. Burlington: Department of Psychiatry, University of Vermont.

Alloway, T. P. (2007). *Automated Working Memory Assessment*. London: Harcourt Assessment.

Ardila, A., Rosselli, M., Matute, E., and Guajardo, G. (2005). The influence of parents' educational level on the development of executive functions. *Developmental Neuropsychology*, 28, 539-560.

Barkley, R. A. (2012). *Barkley Deficits in Executive Functioning Scale* - Children and Adolescents (BDEFS-CA). New York, NY: The Guilford Press.

Barncord, N. (2002). An oral Trail Making Test: a validity investigation. *Archives of Clinical Neuropsychology*, 17, 827-835.

Bishop, T. L. (2011). Relationship between performance-based measures of executive function and the Behavior Rating Inventory of Executive Function (BRIEF), a parent rating measure. *Dissertation Abstracts International: Section B: The Sciences and Engineering*, 72(1-B), 522.

Borys, S. V., Spitz, H. H., and Dorans, B. A. (1982). Tower of Hanoi performance of retarded young adults and nonretarded children as a function of solution length and goal state. *Journal of Experimental Child Psychology*, 33, 87-110.

Brock, L. L., Rimm-Kaufman, S. E. and Nathanson, L. (2009). The contributions of 'hot' and 'cool' executive function to children's academic achievement and learning-related behaviors, and engagement in kindergarten. *Early Childhood Research Quarterly*, 24(3), 337-349.

Burin, D. I., Drake, M., and Harris, P. (2007). Evaluación de la atención [Assessment of Attention]. In D.I. Burin, M. Drake, and P. Harris (Eds.), *Evaluación Neuropsicológica en adultos* [Neuropsychologic assessment in adults] (pp. 146-147) Buenos Aires: Paidós.

Cairos, F. D., and Cammock, J. (1982). *Preliminary norms for the MFF-20.*Unpublished document.

Cairos, E. D., and Cammock, J. (2002). MFF-20. Test de emparejamiento de Figuras Conocidas.[MFF-20. Matching Familiar Figures Test]. Madrid: TEA.

Chan, R., Shum, D., Toulopoulou, T. and Chen, E. (2008). Assessment of executive functions: Review of instruments and identification of critical issues. *Archives of Clinical Neuropsychology* 23, 201-216.

Chevignard, M. P., Catroppa, C., Galvin, J. and Anderson, V. (2010). Development and evaluation of an ecological task to assess executive functioning post childhood TBI: The Children's Cooking Task. Brain Impairment, 11(2), 125–143. doi: http://dx.doi.org/10.1375/brim.11.2.125.

Climent, G., and Bánterla, F. (2011). Aula Nesplora, evaluación ecológica de los procesos atencionales. Manual teórico [Nesplora Classroom, ecological assessment of attentional processes. Theoretical Manual]. Donostia, SP: Nesplora.

Conners, K. C. (2004). *Conners Continuous Performance Test* (2nd ed.). North Tonawanda, NY: Multi-Heath Systems.

Danielsson, H., Henry, L., Messer, D., and Rönnberg, J. (2012). Strengths and weaknesses in executive functioning in children with intellectual disability. *Journal of Research in Developmental Disabilities*, 33(2), 600-607. http://dx.doi.org/10.1016/j.ridd.2011.11.004

Delis, D. C., Kaplan, E., and Kramer, J. (2001). *Delis Kaplan Executive Function System.* San Antonio, TX: The Psychological Corporation.

Diamond, A. (2013). Executive Functions.Annual Review of Psychology, 64, 135-168. doi: 10.1146/annurev-psych-113011-143750.

Diaz-Orueta, U., Garcia-Lopez, C., Crespo-Eguilaz, N., Sanchez-Carpintero, R., Climent, G., and Narbona, J. (2014). AULA virtual reality test as an attention measure: Convergent validity with Conners. Continuous Performance Test. *Child Neuropsychology*, 20(3), 328-342.

Diaz-Orueta, U., Iriarte, Y., Climent, G. and Banterla, F. (2012). AULA: An ecological virtual reality test with distractors for evaluating attention in children and adolescents. *Journal of Virtual Reality*, 5, 1-20.

Dolcos, F., and McCarthy, G. (2006). Brain Systems Mediating Cognitive Interference by Emotional Distraction. *The Journal of Neuroscience*, 26(7), 2072-2079.

Egeland, J., and Fallmyr, Ø. (2010). Confirmatory Factor Analysis of the Behavior Rating Inventory of Executive Function (BRIEF): support for a distinction between emotional and behavioral regulation. *Child Neuropsychology*, 16(4), 326-37. doi: 10.1080/09297041003601462

Emslie, H., Wilson, F., Burden, V., Nimmo-Smith, I., and Wilson, B. A. (2003). *Behavioural Assessment of the Dysexecutive Syndrome for Children (BADSC);* London, UK: Harcourt Assessment/The Psychological Corporation.

Fingerhut, P., Madill, H., Darrah, J., Hodge, M., and Warren, S. (2002). Classroom-based assessment: validation for the school AMPS. *American Journal of Occupational Therapy*, 56(2), 210-213.

García-Molina, A., Tirapu-Ustárroz, J., and y Roig-Rovira, T. (2007). Validez ecológica en la exploración de las funciones ejecutivas [Ecological validity in exploring executive functions]. Anales de Psicología, 23(2), 289-299.

García, T., Rodríguez, C., González-Castro, P., Álvarez, D., Cueli, M., and González-Pienda, J. A. (2013). Executive Functioning in children and adolescents with Attention Deficit Hyperactivity Disorder and Reading Disabilities. *International Journal of Psychology and Psychological Therapy,* 13(2), 179-194.

García, T., González-Castro, P., Rodríguez, C., Álvarez, D., Cueli, M., and Álvarez, L. (2014). Alteraciones del funcionamiento ejecutivo en el Trastorno por Déficit de Atención con Hiperactividad y sus subtipos [Executive functioning deficits in Attention Deficit Hyperactivity Disorder and its subtypes]. *Psicología Educativa*, 20(1), 23-33.

Geurts, H. M., and Marlies, E. U. (2012). Ederly with Autism: Executive Functions and Memory. *Journal of Autism and Developmental Desorders,* 42(5), 665-75. doi: 10.1007/s10803-011-1291-0.

Gioia, G. A., Isquith, P. K., Guy, S., and Kenworthy, L. (2000). *BRIEF: Behavior Rating Inventory of Executive Function professional manual.* Lutz, FL: Psychological Assessment Resources.

Gioia, G. A., Kenworthy, L. and Isquith, P. K. (2010). Executive function in the real world: BRIEF lessons from Mark Ylvisaker. *Journal of Head Trauma Rehabilitation*, 25(6), 433–439. doi: 10.1097/HTR .0b013e3181fbc272

Golden, C. J. (1974). Cognitive, personality, and demographic aspects of the Stroop Color and Word Test. Chapter presented to the annual convention of the Hawaii Psychological Association, Honolulu, Hawaii.

Grant, D. A., and Berg, E. A. A. (1948). A behavioral analysis of degree of reinforcement and ease of shifting to new responses in a Weigel-type card-sorting problem. Journal of Experimental Psychology, 38, 404-411.

Greenberg, M. L. (1996). *Test of Variables of Attention* (TOVA).Los Alamitos, CA: Universal Attention Disorders.

Hale, J. B., Reddy, L. A., Semrud-Clikeman, M., Hain, L. A., Whitaker, J., Morley, J, Lawrence, K., Smith, A., and Jones, N. (2011). Executive Impairments Determines ADHD Medication Response: Implications for Academic Achievement. *Journal of Learning Disabilities*, 55, 196- 212. doi: 10.1177/0022219410391191

Heaton, R. K. (1981). *Wisconsin Card Sorting Test Manual*. Odessa, FL. Psychological Assessment Resource Inc.

Huizinga, H., and Smidts, D. P. (2011). Age-Related Changes in Executive Function: A Normative Study with the Dutch Version of the Behavior Rating Inventory of Executive Function. *Child Neuropsychology*, 17, 51–56. doi: 10.1080/09297049.2010.509715.

Huettel, S. A., Misiureka, J., Jurkowskia, A. J., and McCarthy, G. (2004). Dynamic and strategic aspects of executive processing. *Brain Research* 1000, 78-84. doi: 10.1016/j.brainres.2003.11.041

Iriarte, Y., Diaz-Orueta, U., Cueto, E., Irazustabarrena, P., Flavio Banterla, F., and Climent, G. (2012). AULA—Advanced Virtual Reality Tool for the Assessment of Attention: Normative Study in Spain. *Journal of Attention Disorders,* 20, 1-27. doi: 10.1177/1087054712465335

Kagan, J. (1965). *Matching Familiar Figures Test.* Cambridge, Massachussetts: Harvard University.

Kobayashi, H., and Kobayashi, H. (2007). Study of the behavioural assessment of the dysexecutive syndrome (BADS) in school-aged children. *Journal of Saitama University*, 56, 49-57.

Korzeniowski, C. G. (2011). Desarrollo evolutivo del funcionamiento ejecutivo y su relación con el aprendizaje escolar [Evolutive development of executive functioning and its relationship to learning]. Revista de Psicología, 7(13), 7-26.

Lee, K., Lynn, N., and Fong, S. (2009). The Contributions of Working Memory and Executive Functioning to Problem Representation and Solution Generation in Algebraic Word Problems. *Journal of Educational Psychology,* 101(2), 373–387.

Lee, E. (2011). An exploratory analysis of the ecological validity of a performance-based assessment of attention. *Dissertation Abstracts International: Section B: The Sciences and Engineering*, 71(9-B), 5777.

Lezak, M. D., Howieson D. B., Bigler, E. D., and Tranel, D. (2012). *Neuropsychological assessment 5th edition.* Oxford: Oxford University Press Chapters.

Llorente, A. M., Williams, J., Satz, P., and D´Elia, L. F. (2003). *Children´s Colour Trail Test*. Lutz, FL: Psychological Assessment Resources.

Logan, G. D., Cowan, W. B., and Davis, K. A. (1984). On the Ability to Inhibit Simple and Choice Reaction-Time Responses - a Model and a Method. *Journal of Experimental Psychology-Human Perception and Performance*, 10, 276–291.

Lozano, A., and Ostrosky. (2011). Desarrollo de las Funciones Ejecutivas y de la Corteza Prefrontal [Development of Executive Functions and the Prefrontal Cortex]. Revista Neuropsicología, *Neuropsiquiatría y Neurociencias,* 11(1), 159-172.

Mares, D., McLuckie, A., Schwartz, M., and Saini, M. (2007). Executive function impairments in children with attention-deficit hyperactivity disorder: do they differ between school and home environments? *Canadian Journal of Psychiatry*, 52(8), 527-534.

Martín, R., Hernández, S., Rodríguez, C., García, E., Díaz, A. and Jiménez, J.E. (2012). Datos normativos para el Test de Stroop: patrón de desarrollo de la inhibición y formas alternativas para su evaluación [Normative data for the Stroop Test: Development pattern of inhibition and alternative forms for its assessment]. *European Journal of Education and Psychology*, 5(1), 39-51.

McAuley, T., Chen, S., Goos, L., Schachar, R. and Crosbie, J. (2010). Is the Behavior Rating Inventory of Executive Functions more strongly associated with measures of impairment or executive function? *Journal of the International Neuropsychological Society*, 16(3), 495-505. 10.1017/S1355617710000093.

Mizuno, K., Tanaka, M., Fukuda, S., Imai-Matsumura, K., and Watanabe, Y. (2011). Relationship between cognitive functions and prevalence of fatigue in elementary and junior high school students. *Brain Development*, 33,470-479. doi: 10.1186/1744-9081-7-20.

Pickering, S., and Gathercole, S. E. (2001). *Working Memory Test Battery for Children* (WMTB-C).London: Pearson Assessment.

Reitan, R. M. (1958). Validity of the Trail Making Test as an indicator of organic brain damage. *Perceptual and Motor Skills*, 8, 271-276.

Reynolds, C. R. (2002). *Comprehensive Trail Making Test: Examiner's manual*. Austin, Texas: PRO-E.

Robinson, S., Goddard, L., Dritschel, B., Wisley, M., and Howlin, P. (2009). Executive functions in children with Autism Spectrum Disorders. *Brain and Cognition*, 71, 362–368. doi: 10. 1016/j.bandc.2009.06.007

Rocke, K., Hays, P., Edwards, D. and Berg, C. (2008). Development of a Performance Assessment of Executive Function: The Children's Kitchen Task Assessment. *The American Journal of Occupational Therapy*, 62(5), 528-537.

Rothbart, M. K., Ahadi, S. A., Hershey, K. L., and Fisher, P. (2001). Investigations of temperament at 3–7 years: The Children's Behavior Questionnaire. *Child Development*, 72, 1394–1408.

Salbach-Andrae, H., Klaus Lenz, K., and Lehmkuhl, U. (2009). Patterns of agreement among parent, teacher and youth ratings in a referred sample. *European Psychiatry*, 24(5), 345–351. doi: 10.1016/j.eurpsy.2008.07.008

Schachar, R., Mota, V. L., Logan, G. D., Tannokc, R., and Klim, P. (2000). Confirmation of an inhibitory control deficit in attention-deficit/hyperactivity disorder. *Journal of Abnormal Child Psychology*, 28, 227-236.

Shallice, T. (1982). Specific impairments of planning. Philosophical Transactions of the Royal Society of London. Series B, *Biological Sciences,* 298 (1089), 199-209.

Shimoni, M., Engel-Yeger, B., and Tirosh, E. (2012). Executive dysfunctions among boys with Attention Deficit Hyperactive Disabilities (ADHD): Performance based test and parents report. *Research in Developmental Disabilities,* 33, 858–865.

Silver, C. H., Kolitz-Russell, S., Bordoni, F., and Fairbanks, J. (1993). *The Children´s Executive Functions Scale*. Unpublished rating scale.

Simon, J. R., and Berbaum, K. (1990). Effect of conflicting cues on information processing: The 'Stroop effect' vs. The 'Simon effect'. *Acta Psychologica,* 73(2), 159-170.

Simon, J. R. (1969). Reactions toward the source of stimulation. *Journal of Experimental Psychology*, 81, 174-176. doi: 10.1037/h0027448

Slachevsky, A., Pérez, C., Silva, J., Orellana, J., Prenafeta, M.L., Alegría, P., and Peña, M. (2005). Cortex prefrontal y trastornos del comportamiento. Modelos explicativos y métodos de evaluación [Prefrontal cortex and behavioral disorders. Explanatory models and assessment methods]. *Revista Chilena de Neuropsiquiatría*, 43, 109-121.

Strauss, E., Sherman, E., and Spreen, O. (2006). *A Compendium of Neuropsychological Tests*: Administration, norms, and Commentary (Hardcover). New York: Oxford University Press.

Stroop, J. R. (1935). Studies of interference in serial verbal reactions. *Journal of Experimental Psychology*, 18, 643-622.

Stuss, D. T., and Knight, R. T. (2013). *Principles of Frontal Lobe Function*. New York: Oxford University Press.

Thorell, L. B. and Nyberg, L. (2008). The Childhood Executive Functioning Inventory (CHEXI): A new rating instrument for parents and teachers. *Developmental Neuropsychology*, 33, 536–552. doi: 10.1080/87565640 802101516

Tirapu-Ustárroz, J., García-Molina, A., Luna-Lario, P., Roig-Rovira T., and Pelegrín-Valero, C. (2008). Modelos de funciones y control ejecutivo (II) [Models of executive functions and control (II)]. *Revista de Neurología*, 46(12), 742-750.

Toll, S. W. M., Van der Ven, S. H. G., Kroesbergen, E. H., and Van Luit, J. E. H. (2011). Executive functions as predictors of math learning disabilities. *Journal of Learning Disabilities*, 44(6), 521 – 532.doi: 10.1177/00222194 10387302

Toplak, M. E., Bucciarelli, S. M., Jain, U. and Tannock, R. (2009). Executive functions: performance-based measures and the Behavior Rating of Executive Function (BRIEF) in adolescents with Attention Deficit /Hyperactivity Disorder (ADHD). *Child Neuropsychology*, 15, 53–72. doi: 10.1080/09297040802070929.

Van der Sluis, S., de Jong, P.F., and Van der Leij, A. (2007). Executive functioning in children, and its relations with reasoning, reading, and arithmetic. *Intelligence*, 35, 427-449. doi: 10.1016/j.intell.2006.09.001.

Van der Ven, S. H., Kroesbergen, E. H., Boom, J., and Leseman, P. P. (2013). The structure of executive functions in children: a closer examination of inhibition, shifting, and updating. *British Journal of Developmental Psychology*, 31(1), 70-87. doi: 10.1111/j.2044-835X.2012.02079.x

Van De Voorde, S., Roeyers, H., Verté, S., and Wiersema, J. R. (2010). Working memory, response inhibition, and within-subject variability in children with attention-deficit/hyperactivity disorder or reading disorder. *Journal of Clinical and Experimental Neuropsychology*, 32, 366-79. doi: 10.1080/13803390903066865

Verdejo-García, A., and Bechara, A. (2010). Neuropsychology of Executive Functions. *Psicothema*, 22(2), 227-235.

Wechsler, D. (2003). *Wechsler Intelligence Scale for Children-Fourth Edition*. San Antonio, TX: Psychological Corporation.

Wolosin, S. M., Richardson, M. E., Hennessey, J. G., Denckla, M. B., and Mostofsky, S. H. (2009). Abnormal cerebral cortex structure in children with ADHD. *Human Brain Mapping*, 30(1), 175-184. doi: 10.1002 /hbm.20496.

In: Research Trends in Behavior …
Editor: Miao-Kun Sun
ISBN: 978-1-63485-461-0

Chapter 4

THE BIDIRECTIONAL RELATIONSHIP OF STRESS AND EXECUTIVE FUNCTIONING

Beeta Y. Homaifar[1,3]*, Ph.D., Molly C. Gibian[2], B.A. and Megan L. Petrik, Ph.D.

[1]VISN 19 MIRECC, VA Eastern Colorado Healthcare System, Denver, CO, US

[2]Translational Research Center for TBI and Stress Disorders (TRACTS) and Geriatric Research, Education and Clinical Center (GRECC), VA Boston Healthcare System, Boston, MA, US

[3]Departments of Psychiatry and Physical Medicine and Rehabilitation, University of Colorado School of Medicine, Denver, CO, US

ABSTRACT

The relationship between stress and executive functioning is bidirectional and complex. This manuscript focuses on the relationship of stress and executive functioning with respect to both negative and positive outcomes. First, we highlight the negative impact of stress upon executive functioning. This is followed by a discussion of how executive dysfunction impacts the ability to recover from stress. We then move

* Correspondence and requests for reprints: Beeta Y. Homaifar, PhD, Departments of Psychiatry and Physical Medicine and Rehabilitation, University of Colorado School of Medicine, Anschutz Medical Campus, 1055 Clermont St, Denver, CO 80220, (303) 399-8020 x6119, Email: beeta.homaifar@va.gov

into a discussion of the positive impacts of stress upon executive functioning. Lastly, we discuss how the presence of intact executive functioning can positively impact the process of coping with stress.

Keywords: Stress, Executive Function, Coping

1. Impact of Stress on Executive Functioning: Negative Consequences

The prefrontal cortex, which is largely responsible for the executive functioning processes that underlie the strategies often used to cope with stress (Admon et al., 2009; Raio, Orederu, Palazzolo, Shurick, and Phelps, 2013; Sapolsky, 2004; Taylor, Eisenberger, Saxbe, Lehman, and Lieberman, 2006), is also the brain region most vulnerable to stress (Compass, 2006). Stressors of varying levels of severity can impact cognitive functioning. In the face of acute stressors, there is a neural shift in the brain that "requires the individual to allocate extra resources…this demand for extra resources may reduce processing efficiency and performance" (Galy, Cariou, and Mélan, 2012, p. 269). Specifically, activity in the large-scale network of executive functions is diminished while the networks in control of attentional and threat vigilance are heightened (Hermans et al., 2014). On the other end of the stressor continuum, even mild stress can have deleterious effects on the prefrontal cortex, causing executive functioning to falter (Diamond, 2010, 2013). This section will present research related to negative impact of stress on two frequently studied domains of executive functioning: poor decision making and inflexible thinking.

During times of cognitive and/or emotional stress/overload, healthy adults become overwhelmed at times and make poor decisions (Fraser et al., 2012; Pabst, Schoofs, Pawlikowski, Brand, and Wolf, 2013). Effective decision making is a crucial function in everyday life and requires multiple steps, including holding various aspects of information in memory while considering the benefits and consequences of each option (Diamond, 2013). Thus, decision making requires working memory. In support of this, Nezu and Nezu (2013, p. 10) state "there are limitations in our ability to manipulate large amounts of information in our working memory simultaneously while attempting to solve complex problems or make effective decisions…especially when under stress." Qin et al. (2009) demonstrated that acute laboratory-induced stress (having participants watch short movie clips with extremely aversive content) resulted in reduced working memory as well as executive functioning network activity on whole in healthy adults. Further supporting the link between working memory and stress, Diestel et al. (2013) found that the level of impairment in working memory can be understood as a function of the amount of demand placed on chronically stressed individuals. The authors examined the impact of occupational burnout and task demand on cognitive functioning in nursing home employees. Low and high burnout groups were created via a median split on employees' emotional exhaustion scores. Employees performed two cognitive tasks (N-back and Stroop tasks) measuring working memory under both high and low demand conditions. The high burnout group made more errors and had longer reaction times than the low burnout group, but this difference only occurred when the task demand was high. Thus they suggested that the demand of the task at hand contributes to deterioration in executive functioning even in chronically stressed individuals.

Another component of executive functioning that is impacted by stress is flexible thinking. Sapolsky (2004) notes that whether individuals use problem solving or emotional regulation techniques (or both) to cope with stress depends, in part, on their ability to switch strategies (i.e., engage in flexible thinking) when it is advantageous to do so. Executive functioning underlies the ability to flexibly make optimal use of coping strategies. This is especially relevant in acutely distressed individuals (Homaifar et al., 2012). Homaifar et al. (2012b) note that "Once a crisis has been identified, coping with it requires an ability to flexibly employ various strategies, potentially adapting them to the circumstances until one works" (p. 112). The underlying reasoning behind this is that the predominant use of any one particular coping strategy may be disadvantageous (Cheng and Cheung, 2005).

There has been very little research addressing the relationship between stress and cognitive flexibility (Plessow et al., 2011). In order to examine this relationship, Plessow et al. (2011) asked two groups of individuals to complete a task of selective attention (a control group and a group exposed to an acute stressor immediately prior to the task) and compared the groups on cognitive performance and measures of neuroendocrine stress response. The group exposed to the acute stressor was able to complete the selective attention task, however, did so at the expense of cognitive flexibility. These two groups did not immediately differ in their performance, rather reduced cognitive flexibility and increased salivary cortisol levels were seen in the last segment of the experiment. These results provide evidence that the timing of impairment in executive functioning tasks, such as cognitive flexibility, corresponds with the glucocorticoid response of the hypothalamic-pituitary-adrenal (HPA) axis. Cheng and Cheung (2005) also found that individuals who are less flexible in their use of coping strategies tend to heavily rely on monitoring of threat-related information, which can in turn increase an individual's level of stress and anxiety. This reliance on one type of coping prohibits an individual from flexibly choosing a strategy that would be best suited to dealing with the unique characteristics of various stressors. Ineffective coping with stress is ripe for the opportunity to experience greater or additional stress, thus amplifying the negative impact of stress on executive functioning.

2. Impact of Executive Dysfunction on Stress: Implications for Stress Recovery

Understanding the negative impact of stress upon executive functioning is but one part of the picture. It is also necessary to understand the impact of executive dysfunction upon one's ability to recover from stress. Recovery from stress is often referred to as stress regulation. Stress regulation involves four processes identified by Uchino, Smith, Holt-Lunstad, Campo, and Reblin (2007). Williams, Suchy, and Rau (2009) discuss these processes: exposure, reactivity, recovery, and restoration with respect to their relationship to executive dysfunction. In the following section, brief definitions of each stress regulation process will be provided, followed by how each could be measured. The impact of executive dysfunction on each process will be discussed, and illustrative examples will be offered.

Exposure implies that individuals vary with respect to the degree of stress to which they are exposed (Williams et al., 2009). Measurement of stress exposure often involves determining the frequency and severity of life stressors. Individuals who have difficulty staying on task, organizing, planning, problem-solving, or decision-making are likely to place themselves in situations of frequent and significant stress exposure (Williams et al., 2009). For example, turning in work assignments that are consistently disorganized can invite increased scrutiny and reprimand, thus exposing one to work-related stress.

Reactivity refers to the degree of physiological and emotional response to the stressor (Williams et al., 2009). Measurement of stress reactivity involves objectively determining an individual's physiological reactivity via heart rate, blood pressure, etc. as well as subjectively determining their perception of distress. Objectively, blood pressure reactivity and heart rate variability are affected during times of acute stress (Butler, Wilhelm, and Gross, 2006; Waldstein and Katzel, 2005). Subjectively, individuals who cannot flexibly employ alternate strategies when their primary coping strategy fails are likely to perceive a higher degree of distress than those with no executive functioning impairment. This is likely secondary to their tendency to use the same strategy repeatedly despite evidence that their approach is unsuccessful. These tendencies are especially relevant during crisis situations.

Recovery is the time it takes to recover from stressors (Williams et al., 2009). Measurement of stress recovery involves objectively and subjectively determining the amount of time it requires for an individual's physiological and psychological reactivity to return to baseline, respectively, after a stressor has been withdrawn (Williams et al., 2009). Rumination, defined by Williams et al. (2009) as the tendency to re-imagine a stressor, is hypothesized to play a role in both the physiological and psychological response to stress recovery. Rumination is thought to reduce executive functioning capacity on whole (Watkins and Brown, 2002) and has been hypothesized to interfere with problem-solving (Smith and Alloy, 2009). Some have proposed that rumination is specifically associated with a perseverative cognitive style (Davis and Nolen-Hoeksema, 2000). For example, a study of executive functioning in ruminators compared with nonruminators found that the former committed more perseverative errors on a test of executive functioning (Davis and Nolen-Hoeksema, 2000). Therefore, to the extent that individuals imagine a stressor over and over again during failed attempts to problem-solve about it, this could impact the time it takes for them to recover from the physiological and psychological impacts of stress.

Restoration refers to whether one can re-establish equilibrium on a consistent basis after a stressor has been removed (Williams et al., 2009). Measurement of restoration from stress entails determining whether the individual has returned to baseline levels of allostatic load consistently (Williams et al., 2009). Restorative processes include things such as healthy sleep patterns. Executive functioning can affect restoration in that those with impairments in insight may lack the awareness that restoration is necessary in the first place. This can translate into individuals who may not be aware that getting back to healthy sleep patterns, after a period of stress that resulted in poor sleep, is necessary. Even if an individual's insight is functioning well, impairments in decision making can prevent them from optimally engaging in restoration activities. This can translate into individuals who know they need to return to healthy sleep patterns after a period of stress that resulted in poor sleep, yet they engage in poor sleep hygiene, which can impede restorative sleep.

3. Impact of Stress on Executive Functioning: Positive Consequences

In order to successfully manage and recover from a stressful experience, an individual must often effectively employ various executive functions. This section will describe relevant research in which stress has been shown to improve executive function. Parker et al. (2004) examined stress inoculation prospectively in a primate population by demonstrating that laboratory-induced mild early life stress strengthened resistance to subsequent stressors. Monkeys exposed to moderate, intermittent stress demonstrated less anxiety and decreased stress hormone levels in subsequent novel stressful environments as compared to monkeys without prior stress experiences. Parker et al. (2005) expanded on those findings by examining the effect of stress inoculation on later cognitive control. Specifically, they found that response inhibition errors were lower in primates who had experienced stress inoculation, in addition to improved emotional and neuroendocrine stress resistance.

In adult humans, neuropsychological studies have shown that exposure to some stress is more beneficial than exposure to no stress or high stress. Henderson, Snyder, Gupta, and Banich (2012) found that exposure to controllable, moderate levels of laboratory-induced stress (via loud noise and feedback regarding accuracy of performance) benefited performance on a test of general executive functioning. In contrast, exposure to uncontrollable laboratory-induced stress, or having an extreme reaction to stress, harmed performance. They suggested that individuals should expose themselves to the types of stress that promote the most enhanced functioning possible. Research by Maier and Watkins (2010) would also recommend exposure to stress that is controllable. They found that exposure to a controllable stressor initiated activation of the ventral medial prefrontal cortex, which mediated and inhibited stress-responsive limbic and brainstem structures. The same activation (and accompanying stress resistance) occurred in subsequent trials, even when the stressor was uncontrollable. In line with this, Stawski, Almeida, Lachman, Tun, and Rosnick (2010) found that healthy adults who demonstrated the most optimal performance on measures of executive functioning, including problem-solving, had greater exposure and less negative reactions to daily stressors. Thus, their findings provide ecological validity to the idea that exposure to stress can positively impact executive functioning. Another study found that acute stress can positively affect decision-making, but in a time-dependent manner. Performance on a task of decision-making at time points within 5 or 18 minutes of stress exposure, at the highest levels of sympathetic nervous system activation, was associated with less risky decision-making. However, performance on the same task of decision-making within 28 minutes of stress exposure, at the peak of hypothalamic-pituitary-adrenal activity, was associated with more risky decision-making (Pabst, Brand, and Wolf, 2013). These studies suggest that some exposure to stress, particularly if it is before cortisol reaches its peak, may have neuro-psychological benefits in humans.

Other research indicates that a stressful situation may engage more efficient processes with corresponding changes in neural activation patterns. Gathmann et al. (2014) found that stressful situations can initiate a switch to parallel, lower-resource processes in the context of a dual task design. In this study, the additional stress of a second task requiring greater working memory load did not cause a decrease in behavioral performance, but rather caused an increase in prefrontal activation. Essentially, more executive resources were necessary in order to navigate the switch from serial to parallel processing. Similarly, Jaeggi et al. (2007) found that the brains of high performers respond differently than low performers when performing a task of increasing working memory capacity. High performers displayed activation patterns reflecting more efficient and relaxed processing, while low performers had larger load-dependent activation increases in key cortical areas (dorsolateral prefrontal cortex). Qualitatively, high performers reported less explicit strategy use and reported relying more on intuitive processes. Low performers reported using many strategies and switched strategies often as their performance declined. This study suggests that compensatory and effortful prefrontal activation in low performers may unnecessarily draw cognitive resources away from automatic systems capable of more efficient processing. High performers "kept their cool," allowing their functioning to remain intact, resourceful, and adaptive.

4. Impact of Executive Functioning on Stress: Implications for Coping

In order to be resilient in the face of stressors, one must employ effective coping strategies that often involve executive functioning. One such valuable coping strategy is cognitive reappraisal. Cognitive reappraisal is the act of redefining a negative experience (Rutter, 2006). For example, suppose an individual experiences a stressor or adverse event and wishes to cope via reappraising the situation in a positive light, thereby increasing the possibility of a beneficial outcome. Cognitive reappraisal of the situation would involve working memory in that the individual must be able to think about the problem and, while holding information about the problem in memory, change his/her perspective about it (Compass, 2006). Research has shown that individuals can experience beneficial psychological changes after significant negative life events when they are able to perceive some benefit as a consequence (McAdams, Reynolds, Lewis, Patten, and Bowman, 2013; Taylor, Kemeny, Reed, Bower, and Gruenewald, 2000; Tedeschi and Calhoun, 1996). The ability to change one's perspective about a negative event can foster a turning point in one's life. Turning points involve finding meaning in adverse events. Operationally, finding meaning can be broadly defined as "a major shift in values, priorities, or perspectives," often in response to a loss or some other negative event (Taylor et al., 2000, p. 105). The effortful process of finding meaning in adverse life events requires continual executive function (reappraisal). In order to understand how individuals derive meaning at a turning point, we must understand more about their executive functioning.

There remains, however, a dearth of research with respect to understanding the process of finding meaning after negative life events (McMackin, Newman, Fogler, and Keane, 2012). McAdams et al. (2013) examined the relationship of executive functioning and meaning in the context of a turning point, although indirectly. Interviews with college-aged and middle-aged adults about their life stories showed that those who were highly generative reported more positive turning points (after a negative event) than less generative adults. Generativity was measured via several instruments that assessed participants' concern for having a positive effect on the next generation, and the extent to which participants engaged in volitional behavior. While generativity was not defined as a neuropsychological construct, it is widely accepted that generativity (i.e., volitional behavior) is a crucial part of intact executive functioning (Lezak, Howieson, and Loring, 2004).

Mohlman and Gorman (2005) suggest that executive abilities are integral to success in cognitive behavior therapy (CBT). They measured executive functioning before and after CBT in a population of older adults and found that those with persistent executive dysfunction did not respond to CBT treatment for generalized anxiety disorder. In contrast, those with adequate executive abilities responded well to CBT and reported greater emotional benefit as a result of the therapy. Johnco, Wuthrich, and Rapee (2014) expanded on these findings in older adults by targeting cognitive flexibility. These researchers found that better initial cognitive flexibility was related to better adaptation and use of cognitive restructuring tools learned in therapy. Those with poor initial cognitive flexibility reported less benefit from the cognitive restructuring strategies. As such, an individual's presenting level of cognitive function (or dysfunction), particularly in the executive realm, should be taken into account when initiating cognitive therapy.

Cognitive reappraisal is also beneficial when employed in situations of acute stress in order to mitigate physiological stress responses. During a stressful experience, an individual is interpreting a great deal of incoming information. They must evaluate the environment, weigh the relative demands of the situation with their perceived personal resources, and manage their physiological response. Each of these processes involves resourceful executive functioning. Jamieson, Mendes, and Nock (2013) focus on arousal reappraisal, in which individuals are encouraged to interpret their physiological stress response as a resource that aids performance. This type of reappraisal "is not aimed at eliminating or dampening stress arousal but instead focuses on changing the type of stress response" (p. 53). These researchers cite numerous studies in which participants who positively reinterpreted their bodily cues displayed more adaptive physiological and psychological responses (Jamieson et al., 2012; Jamieson et al., 2013b; Jamieson et al., 2010). The improvements included altered cardiovascular function (decreased vasoconstriction and greater cardiac output), decreased vigilance, reduced attentional bias, and a faster return to baseline physiological levels. In sum, favorable evaluation of physical sensations allowed participants to use their heightened stress response to facilitate a beneficial outcome. In a similar vein, Harvey, Nathens, Bandiera, and LeBlanc (2010) also described the effects of cognitive appraisal on physiological responses while measuring appraisal as the subjective ratio of situational demands to available resources. In a medical trauma scenario, trainees who interpreted a high stress scenario as a 'threat' (in which demands of the situation exceeded personal resources) had greater HPA axis activation. The more extreme their 'threat' appraisals, the greater their cortisol levels.

Therefore, in order to improve performance and reduce physiological stress, interventions for acute stress scenarios could focus on the analysis of relative resources and demands of the situation, in order to reappraise the situation as a 'challenge' rather than a 'threat.'

Conclusion

It is clear that the relationship between stress and executive functioning is bidirectional and complex, thus warranting further research. Longitudinal studies that measure and track executive functioning and exposure to stress over time may unearth potential mechanisms by which these constructs are affected. Cross-sectional studies of potential moderators and/or mediators may also be helpful in this regard.

References

Admon, R., Lubin, G., Stern, O., Rosenberg, K., Sela, L., Ben-Ami, H., and Hendler, T. (2009). Human vulnerability to stress depends on amygdala's predisposition and hippocampal plasticity. *Proceedings on the National Academy of Sciences,* 106 (33), 14120-14125.

Bonanno, G. A. (2004). Loss, trauma, and human resilience: Have we underestimated the human capacity to thrive after extremely aversive events? *American Psychologist*, 59, 20–28.

Butler, E. A., Wilhelm, F. H., and Gross, J. J. (2006). Respiratory sinus arrhythmia, emotion, and emotion regulation during social interaction. *Psychophysiology,* 43, 612-622.

Cheng, C., and Cheung, M. W. (2005). Cognitive processes underlying coping flexibility: Differentiation and integration. *Journal of personality*, 73(4), 859-886.

Compass, B. (2006). Psychobiological processes of stress and coping: Implications for resilience in children and adolescents: Comments on the papers of Romeo and McEwen and Fisher et al. *Annals of New York Academy of Sciences,* 1094, 226-234.

Davis, R. N., and Nolen-Hoeksema, S. (2000). Cognitive inflexibility among ruminators and nonruminators. *Cognitive Therapy and Research*, 24, 699–711. doi:10.1023/A:1005591412406

Diamond, A. (2010, May). What do we know about child development and the brain that can help promote resilience and help more children be strong and joyful? Paper Presented at the Annual International Trauma Conference, Boston, MA.

Diamond, A. (2013). Executive functions. *Annual review of psychology*, 64, 135-168.

Diestel, S., Cosmar, M., and Schmidt, K. H. (2013). Burnout and impaired cognitive functioning: The role of executive control in the performance of cognitive tasks. *Work and Stress*, 27(2), 164-180.

Dienstbier, R.A. (1989). Arousal and physiological toughness: Implications for mental and physical health. *Psychological Review*, 96, 84-100.

Dunn, B. D., Dalgleish, T., and Lawrence, A. D. (2006). The somatic marker hypothesis: A critical evaluation. *Neuroscience and Biobehavioral Reviews,* 30, 239–271. doi:10.1016/j.neubiorev.2005.07.001

D'Zurilla, T. J., Nezu, A. M., Maydeu-Olivares, A. (2002). Social Problem-Solving Inventory Revised (SPSI-R): *Technical Manual.* North Tonawanda, NY: Multi-Health Systems, Inc.

Fellows, L. K., and Farah, M. J. (2005). Different underlying impairments in decision-making following ventromedial and dorsolateral frontal lobe damage in humans. Cerebral Cortex, 15, 58–63. doi:10.1093/cercor /bhh108

Fraser, K., Ma, I., Teteris, E., Baxter, H., Wright, B., and McLaughlin, K. (2012). Emotion, cognitive load and learning outcomes during simulation training. *Medical Education*, 46(11), 1055-1062.

Galy, E., Cariou, M., and Mélan, C. (2012). What is the relationship between mental workload factors and cognitive load types? International Journal of *Psychophysiology,* 83(3), 269-275.

Gathmann, B., Schulte, F. P., Maderwald, S., Pawlikowski, M., Starcke, K., Schäfer, L. C., Schöler, T., Wolf, O.T., and Brand, M. (2014). Stress and decision making: Neural correlates of the interaction between stress, executive functions, and decision making under risk. *Experimental brain research,* 232(3), 957-973.

Harvey, A., Nathens, A., Bandiera, G., and LeBlanc, V. (2010). Threat and challenge: Cognitive appraisal and stress responses in simulated trauma recuscitations. *Medical Education*, 44, 587-594. doi:10.1111/j.1365-2923.2010.03634.x

Henderson, R.K., Snyder, H.R., Gupta, T., and Banich, M.T. (2012). When does stress help or harm? The effects of stress controllability and subjective stress response on Stroop performance. *Frontiers in Psychology,* 3(17). doi: 10.3389/fpsyg.2012.00179. eCollection 2012.

Hermans, E. J., Henckens, M. J., Joëls, M., and Fernández, G. (2014). Dynamic adaptation of large-scale brain networks in response to acute stressors. *Trends in Neurosciences*, 37(6), 304-314.

Homaifar, B.Y., Bahraini, N., Silverman, M., and Brenner, L.A. (2012). Executive functioning as a component of suicide risk assessment: Clarifying its role in standard clinical applications. *Journal of Mental Health Counseling,* 34(2), 110-120.

Jaeggi, S.M., Buschkuehl, M., Etienne, A., Ozdoba, C., Perrig, W.J., and Nirkko, A.C. (2007). On how high performers keep cool brains in situations of cognitive overload. *Cognitive, Affective, and Behavioral Neuroscience*, 7(2), 75-89.

Jamieson, J.P., Mendes, W.B., Blackstock, E., and Schmader, T. (2010). Turning the knots in your stomach into bows: Reappraising arousal improves performance on the GRE. *Journal of Experimental Social Psychology,* 46, 208-212.

Jamieson, J.P., Mendes, W.B., and Nock, M.K. (2013). Improving acute stress responses: The power of reappraisal. *Current Directions in Psychological Science,* 22(1), 51-56. doi:10.1177/0963721412461500.

Jamieson, J.P., Nock, M.K. and Mendes, W.B. (2013b). Changing the conceptualization of stress improves affective and physiological outcomes in social anxiety disorder. *Clinical Psychological Science*, 1(4), 363-374. doi: 10.1177/2167702613482119.

Jamieson, J.P., Nick, M.K., and Mendes, W.B. (2012). Mind over matter: Reappraising arousal improves cardiovascular and cognitive responses to stress. *Journal of Experimental Psychology: General*, 141, 417-422.

Johnco, C., Wuthrich, V.M., and Rapee, R.M. (2014). The influence of cognitive flexibility on treatment outcome and cognitive restructuring skill acquisition during cognitive behavioural treatment for anxiety and depression in older adults: Results of a pilot study. *Behavior Research and Therapy,* 57, 55-64. doi: http://dx.doi.org/10.1016/j.brat.2014.04.005.

Kray, L. J., George, L. G., Liljenquist, K. A., Galinsky, A. D., Tetlock, P. E., and Rose, N. J. (2010). From what might have been to what must have been: Counterfactual thinking creates meaning. *Journal of Personality and Social Psychology,* 98(1), 106-118.

Lezak, M. D., Howieson, D. B., and Loring, D. W. (2004). *Neuropsychological assessment* (4th ed.). New York, NY: Oxford University Press.

Maier, S.F., and Watkins, L.R. (2010). Role of the medial prefrontal cortex in coping and resilience. *Brain Research*, 1355, 52-60. doi:10.1016 /j.brainres.2010.08.039.

McAdams, D. P., Reynolds, J., Lewis, M., Patten, A. H., and Bowman, P. J. (2013). When bad things turn good and good things turn bad: Sequences of redemption and contamination in life narrative and their relation to psychosocial adaptation in midlife adults and students. *Personality and Social Psychology Bulletin,* 27, 472-83.

McMackin, R. A., Newman, E., Fogler, J. M., and Keane, T. M. (Eds.). (2012). *Trauma therapy in context: The science and craft of evidence-based practice.* Washington, DC: American Psychological Association.

Mohlman, J., and Gorman, J.M. (2004). The role of executive functioning in CBT: a pilot study with anxious older adults. *Behaviour Research and Therapy*, 43, 447-465. doi:10.1016/j.brat.2004.03.007.

Nezu, A. M., and Nezu, C. M. (2013). Problem-solving strategies. In D. Dozois (Vol. Ed.), *The Wiley handbook of cognitive behavioral therapy: Part One, General strategies* (pp. 1-18). New York: Wiley.

Pabst, S., Brand, M., and Wolf, O. T. (2013). Stress and decision making: A few minutes make all the difference. *Behavior and Brain Research*, 250, 39-45. doi: 10.1016/j.bbr.2013.04.046.

Pabst, S., Schoofs, D., Pawlikowski, M., Brand, M., and Wolf, O. T. (2013). Paradoxical effects of stress and an executive task on decisions under risk. *Behavioral Neuroscience*, 127(3), 369-79. doi: 10.1037/a0032334.

Parker, K.J. Buckmaster, C.L., Justus, K.R., Schatzberg, A.F., and Lyons, D.M. (2005). Mild early life stress enhances prefrontal-dependent response inhibition in monkeys. *Journal of Biological Psychiatry*, 57, 848-855. doi;10.1016/j.biopsych.2004,12.024.

Parker, K.J., Buckmaster, C.L., Schatzberg, A.F., and Lyons, D.M. (2004). Prospective investigation of stress inoculation in young monkeys. *Archives of General Psychiatry*, 61, 933-941.

Plessow, F., Rischer, R., Kirschbaum, C., and Goschke, T. (2011). Inflexibly focused under stress: Acute psychosocial stress increases shielding of action goals at the expense of reduced cognitive flexibility with increasing time lag to the stressor. *Journal of Cognitive Neuroscience*, 23(11), 3218-3227.

Qin, S., Hermans, E. J., van Marle, H. J. F., Luo, J., and Fernandez, G. (2009). Acute psychological stress reduces working memory-related activity in the dorsolateral prefrontal cortex. *Biological Psychiatry*, 66, 25-32.

Raio, C. M., Orederu, T. A., Palazzolo, L., Shurick, A. A., and Phelps, E. A. (2013). Cognitive emotion regulation fails the stress test. *Proceedings of the National Academy of Sciences,* 110(37), 15139-44. doi: 10.1073/pnas.1305706110.

Rutter, M. (2006). Implications of resilience concepts for scientific understanding. *Annals of the New York Academy of Sciences*, 1094, 1–12.

Sapolsky, R. M. (2004). *Why zebras don't get ulcers*, 3rd edition. New York: W. H. Freeman.

Smith, J. M., and Alloy, L. B. (2009). A roadmap to rumination: A review of the definition, assessment, and conceptualization of this multifaceted construct. *Clinical Psychology Review*, 29, 116–128. doi:S0272-7358(08)00141-4[pii]10.1016/j.cpr.2008.10.003

Stawski, R.S., Almeida, D. M., Lachman, M.E., Tun, P.A., and Rosnick, C.B. (2010). Fluid cognitive ability is associated with greater exposure and smaller reactions to daily stressors. *Psychology of Aging*, 25(2), 330-42. doi: 10.1037/a0018246.

Taylor, S. E., Eisenberger, N. I., Saxbe, D., Lehman, B. J., and Lieberman, M. D. (2006). Neural responses to emotional stimuli are associated with childhood family stress. *Biological Psychiatry*, 60, 296-301.

Taylor, S. E., Kemeny, M. E., Reed, G. M., Bower, J. E., and Gruenewald, T. L. (2000). *Psychological resources, positive illusions, and health. American Psychologist*, 55(1), 99-109.

Tedeschi, R.G. and Calhoun, L.G. (1996). The Posttraumatic Growth Inventory: Measuring the positive legacy of trauma. *Journal of Traumatic Stress*, 9(3), 455-471.

Uchino, B.N., Smith, T.W., Holt-Lunstad, J., Campo, R., and Reblin, M. (2007). Stress and Illness. In Cacioppo, J. T and Tassinary, L. G. (Eds.), *Handbook of Psychophysiology* (pp. 608-632). New York, NY: Cambridge University Press.

Waldstein, S. R., Katzel, L. I. Stress-induced blood pressure reactivity and cognitive function. *Neurology*, 64, 1746-1749.

Watkins, E., and Brown, R. G. (2002). Rumination and executive function in depression: An experimental study. *Journal of Neurology, Neurosurgery, and Psychiatry*, 72, 400–402.

Williams, P.G., Suchy, Y., and Rau, H.K. (2009). Individual differences in executive functioning: Implications for stress regulation. *Annals of Behavioral Medicine*, 37, 126-140.

In: Research Trends in Behavior ...
Editor: Miao-Kun Sun
ISBN: 978-1-63485-461-0

Chapter 5

NEURAL CORRELATES OF EMOTION REGULATION: AN FMRI STUDY OF BIG PICTURE REAPPRAISAL

Crystal Lantrip, Ph.D. [1*]***, Stephanie Rude, Ph.D.*** [2] ***and Greg Allen, Ph.D.*** [3]

[1]Neuropsychology Program, Department of Psychiatry, Geisel School of Medicine at Dartmouth, Lebanon, NH, US
[2]Counseling Psychology Program, University of Texas at Austin, Austin, TX, US
[3]School Psychology Program, University of Texas at Austin, Austin, TX, US

ABSTRACT

In neuroimaging paradigms, reappraisal has received considerable attention as an effective emotion regulation strategy but most studies have instructed participants to 'reappraise' impersonal emotion-evoking stimuli as opposed to real-life events and have not given specific guidance regarding how to reappraise. Big picture reappraisal is a specific emotion regulation strategy that offers a way of managing distress aiming

* Correspondence and requests for reprints: Crystal Lantrip, Ph.D., Neuropsychology Program, Department of Psychiatry, Geisel School of Medicine at Dartmouth, One Medical Center Drive, Lebanon, NH 03756-0001; E-mail: crystal.lantrip@hitchcock.org

to promote acceptance and cognitive coping. Big picture reappraisal instructions resulted in activation in bilateral superior parietal lobe, associated with abstraction, as well as areas associated with cognitive control of emotion (orbital frontal cortex, medial prefrontal cortex, lobule VI cerebellum) when compared to distraction and rumination instructions.

Keywords: emotion regulation, neuroimaging, reappraisal

1. INTRODUCTION

The past decade has witnessed an upsurge of interest in the role of emotion regulation strategies in maintaining personal well-being. Reappraisal, which involves changing thoughts about a situation in order to decrease the emotional impact (Gross, 2002), appears to be an effective emotion regulation strategy. This claim is supported by findings that instructions to reappraise result in more positive mood and lower rumination (Kross, Davidson, Weber, and Ochsner, 2009; Ray et al., 2005; Richards and Gross, 2000), and by findings of a positive relationship between self-reported trait reappraisal and indicators of well-being ranging from self-report measures of depression (e.g., Gross and John, 2003; Joorman and Gotlib, 2010) to downregulation of amygdala activity (Ochsner and Gross, 2008).

Given the effectiveness of reappraisal as an emotion regulation strategy, there has been interest in its neurological underpinnings. Research has found that a positive relationship exists between use of reappraisal and executive functioning. For example, self-reported trait reappraisal was correlated with greater self-reported executive functions in daily life in a sample of healthy adolescents and with good performance on task-based emotion regulation paradigms (Gyurak et al., 2009; Lantrip, Isquith, Koven, Welsh and Roth, 2014).

There have also been a number of functional magnetic resonance imaging (fMRI) studies of reappraisal, which have been reviewed by Ochsner, Silvers, and Buhle (2012). Results suggest that posterior and lateral prefrontal and parietal cortex activation (implicated in working memory, selective attention, and inhibition), are strongly associated with the downregulation of negative affect and amygdala deactivation. Dorsal anterior cingulate cortex has been implicated in performance monitoring that may help track the extent to which one's current reappraisal is changing emotional responses in the intended way

(Thompson-Schill, Bedny, and Goldberg, 2005). Dorsal medial prefrontal cortex has also been associated with downregulation of negative affect to a lesser degree, but has been discussed more with regard to positive or negative self-referential thinking (Olsson and Ochsner, 2008).

Despite promising evidence for the usefulness of reappraisal as an emotion regulation strategy, our understanding is limited by inadequate specification of the reappraisal process and artificial laboratory paradigms: Most studies have either correlated Gross and John's (2003) short reappraisal scale (e.g., "I change my thinking as a way to change my mood") with measures of wellbeing, or have manipulated reappraisal in the lab with direct instructions to simply "reappraise," "decrease negative affect," or be more analytical (e.g., analyze a photo) when presented with emotional stimuli. The artificial nature of the emotional stimuli used (typically IAPS pictures or emotional videos) and of the vaguely specified reappraisal strategies seriously limits ecological validity of these studies. Using reappraisal to alter one's emotional response to a picture presented in the lab is fundamentally different from using it in an actual life situation, and strategies that work well in the former situation might be ineffective or even counterproductive in real-life.

Only recently have researchers begun to experimentally investigate specific reappraisal strategies, doing so in naturalistic contexts. One example is Rude and colleagues' (e.g., Rude et al., 2013) work on thinking about distressing experiences from an expanded perspective. These researchers have described big picture appraisal as maintaining awareness of how a distressing event fits into larger contexts, including that of an expanded time frame, the multiple domains of one's life, and the broader human context. Rude, Mazzetti, Pal, and Stauble (2011) presented evidence that adopting such a perspective produced lower symptoms of rumination and depression for college students contemplating a recent social rejection. In this study, Rude and colleagues found that participants experienced lower levels of rumination after receiving an experimental big picture intervention (writing about how they would feel about the experience in 1-2 years, how their responses were similar to those of other people, and how a neutral observer might describe the situation) as compared to those instructed to explore the reasons for the event (e.g., Why do you think this happened?) or those not instructed to write.

Compelling evidence for the benefits of an expanded perspective has also been reported by Schartau, Dalgleish, and Dunn (2009) with regard to their construct of perspective broadening, and by Kross, Ayduk, and their colleagues with regard to their construct of self-distancing (Ayduk and Kross, 2010; Kross and Ayduk, 2008; Kross, Gard, Deldin, Clifton, and Ayduk,

2012). Adopting an expanded, self-distanced perspective has been shown to be associated not only with better mood, lower levels of rumination, and reframed understanding of problems, but also greater cognitive flexibility and problem-solving behavior (Ayduk and Kross, 2010). These research programs, while varying in the particular definitions and paradigms used, have produced evidence of psychological benefits stemming from induction of a larger or more distanced perspective on adversity.

The above research has provided support for the utility of reappraising by adopting an expanded perspective, but the neurological underpinnings of these specific appraisal strategies have not yet received much attention. Given the apparent benefits of regulating emotions by expanding one's perspective, the question arises, what are the cognitive demands and neural correlates of perspective broadening strategies applied in naturalistic situations?

We found only one study that examined reappraisal using naturalistic, self-relevant stimuli to evoke emotion. Kross, Davidson, Weber, and Ochsner (2009), asked 16 healthy participants to reflect on negative autobiographical experiences to induce emotion. In one reappraisal condition, participants were instructed to "accept" feelings--to recognize that their feelings "were passing mental events that were psychologically distant from the self and did not control them," (Kross, Davidson, Weber, and Ochsner, 2009 [pp. 361] for quote).

In a second, "analyze" reappraisal condition, participants were asked to objectively analyze the causes and reasons underlying their feelings. A "feel" condition in which participants were instructed to simply focus on naturally flowing feelings comprised a comparison condition.

Overall, this study found that in a more ecologically valid paradigm, reappraisal instructions were associated with activation in regions previously associated with reappraisal in laboratory paradigms (i.e., left prefrontal cortex activity in response to all three conditions (feel, analyze, and accept), as well as subgenual anterior cingulate and medial prefrontal cortex activation that was highest in response to the feel strategy and lower for the accept strategy, and in accept versus feel, caudate, medial prefrontal cortex, and superior parietal gyrus were active). These results lend credibility to using autobiographical prompts to elicit emotion.

The purpose of the current paper was to determine whether big picture thinking would show neural activation patterns similar to those observed in prior reappraisal research. In addition, we sought to discover whether the high demand of big picture thinking for abstraction would lead to a unique neural signature.

We recruited women experiencing continuing distress about a social rejection and, after instructing them to bring their rejection experience to mind, induced them to employ either a big picture perspective (e.g., "think about how all your past feelings changed with time"), a rumination perspective (e.g., "think about why things turn out the way they do") or a distraction condition (e.g., "focus fully on the layout of a typical classroom"). Mood ratings, active controls (counting backwards), and inactive controls (visual fixation) were interspersed with condition prompts.

We expected that using big picture thinking to reappraise an actual distressing event would likely involve the neurocircuitry observed in previous reappraisal paradigms associated with cognitive control consistent with the theory (Gross, 2002) and research (e.g., Ray et al., 2005) demonstrating that reappraisal requires recruitment of these regions. Specifically the dorsal lateral prefrontal cortex (dlPFC) and inferior parietal lobe (Gross, 2002; Ochsner, Silvers, and Buhle, 2012) were expected to be activated by big picture thinking instructions.

Big picture reappraisal was hypothesized to also result in dorsal medial PFC (dmPFC) activation as compared to distraction, based on research showing this region to be associated not only with cognitive control of emotion, but self-referential thinking (e.g., Ray et al., 2005). The distraction manipulation was designed to produce non self-referential thinking.

In addition, big picture thinking was expected to have its own neural "signature" in that it is theorized to require high levels of abstraction. Abstract thinking involves mentally manipulating information, drawing on working memory, and making generalizations from more specific scenarios /information. Working memory is thought to be localized to the superior parietal lobe (Koenigs, Barbey, Postle, and Grafman, 2009); hence, we hypothesized that activation of this area would be produced by big picture thinking instructions.

Further, there has been a growing body of evidence to suggest that the cerebellum has a primary role in the integrating cognition and emotion (Schmanmann and Sherman, 1998); accordingly, we also hypothesized that activation of the cerebellum would accompany big picture thinking. The above-described activation patterns were expected to occur in comparison to distraction and rumination, as well as an active control involving mental arithmetic.

Regarding possible mood effects of the manipulations, distraction was expected to result in slightly more positive mood than rumination during the task. While big picture thinking is expected to lead to better emotional resolution in the long run, it was not clear whether differences would be observed across the short span of each appraisal induction. Hence, no specific hypotheses were posed regarding mood differences between big picture thinking and the other conditions.

2. Methods

2.1. Sample

Female, right-handed community members from the Central Texas area (N=28; mean age = 25.83, standard deviation = 9.28; Caucasian = 48%, Asian descent = 24%, Hispanic/Latina = 20%, African American = 8%) were recruited from online advertisements, local media, and posted flyers. Flyers stated that participants needed to have a recent social rejection experience in order to be study-eligible and compensation was available for participation. Prior to study entry, potential participants underwent a phone screening to gather information regarding demographics, MRI safety, diagnostic and medication status, and recent rejection history. Participants were included if they answered in the affirmative to the question "have you experienced a rejection experience in the past six months that still bothers you?" and the situation was interpersonal in nature (e.g., romantic breakup, argument with a friend). Participants were excluded from the study if they reported having a current DSM-IV-TR diagnosis by a mental health professional, were currently in therapy, or taking psychiatric medications. The data from two participants were not useable due to unexpected problems with the scanner and one person discontinued participation after becoming claustrophobic in the scanner making the analysis total N=25.

2.2. Conditions and Design

The study examined the effects of prompting participants to reflect upon a recent social rejection under three conditions: Big Picture Reappraisal, Distraction, and Rumination. Each run maintained the same order and timing of stimuli and included a full set of nine prompts for one of the three conditions. Each run was initiated with three prompts guiding the participant to think about their rejection experience in an attempt to prime the experience of rejection, followed by a prompt to rate mood. Next a series of nine condition-specific prompts was administered in three sets of three. Prompts for the Big Picture Reappraisal condition were developed based on Rude (2013) and Rude et al. (2011). The three sets of prompts (each set preceded by the instruction: "Think about…") for the Big Picture Reappraisal condition were: 1) "How all moods come and go with time," "How this one moment fits into your whole life," "How all your past feelings changed with time;" (2) "How you have both good times and bad times," "How important this will seem when you look back on it," "How others have had similar things happen;" (3) "The way you will view this several years from now," "How your feelings are like those of others," "How every person experiences highs and lows)."

Prompts and instructions for the Rumination and Distraction conditions were drawn from Nolen-Hoeksema (S. Nolen-Hoeksema, personal communication, March 23, 2009). The three sets of prompts (each set preceded by the instruction: "Think about…") for the Rumination condition were: 1) What it would be like if your present feelings lasted, Why things turn out the way they do, Trying to understand your feelings, 2) What people notice about your personality, How quick/slow your thinking is right now, Trying to understand who you are, 3) Why you turned out this way, Why you react the way you do, How hopeful/hopeless you are feeling. The three sets of prompts (each set preceded by the instruction: "Focus your attention fully on…") for the Distraction condition were: 1) A boat slowly crossing the Atlantic, The layout of a typical classroom, The shape of a large black umbrella, 2) Movement of an electric fan on a warm day, Raindrops sliding down a windowpane, A double decker bus driving down a street, 3) The expression on the face of the Mona Lisa, Two birds sitting on a tree branch, The shadow of a stop sign. Each set of condition-specific prompts was interspersed with mood ratings (ranging from 1 (negative) to 5 (positive) indicated using a 5-button response box with the dominant hand) and active and inactive controls. The specific sequence (repeated three times per run) was: three sequential condition-specific prompts, mood rating, counting backwards (active control), mood rating, visual fixation crosshairs (inactive control), and another mood rating. Each participant completed two of the three possible runs, determined through random assignment. Participants rested for approximately one minute between runs. Each run took approximately seven minutes. The runs were programmed using DMDX Software (Forster and Forster, 2003).

2.3. Imaging Assessment and fMRI Data Acquisition

Scanning was performed on a whole body 3T GE MRI scanner with an 8 channel phase array head coil. The scanning protocol involved a collection of a localizer, shimming routines, a T1-weighted high-resolution structural scan, and then the functional MRI data collection. The structural scan used was one 3D SPGR volume acquisition, with 1.4 mm thick axial slices for a total of 134 slices (Flip=10 degrees, TR=9.7 ms, TE=4 ms, TI=20 ms, TD=0 ms, FOV=25 cm, Matrix=256X256, NEX=1).

Functional MRI data were acquired while participants completed the emotion regulation task. MR images were collected utilizing whole head coverage with slice orientation to reduce artifact (approximately 20 degrees off the AC-PC plane, TR = 2 sec., TE = 23 msec., 31 axial slices oriented for best whole head coverage, acquisition voxel size = 3.125 X 3.125 X 3 mm with a .3 mm inter-slice gap). A multiecho GRAPPA parallel imaging EPI sequence was used to optimize BOLD signal in regions susceptible to artifact. Stimuli were viewed through a back projection screen and a mirror mounted on the top of the head coil. Responses were collected with 5 button MR compatible optical transmission devices that were held in one hand. Head motion was minimized with foam inserts.

2.3.1. fMRI Analysis

Imaging data were analyzed in a multistage process using FEAT (fMRI Expert Analysis Tool; FMRIB, Oxford, United Kingdom, http://www.fmrib.ox.ac.uk/fsl). Preprocessing was conducted along standard procedures in FEAT. Raw, unprocessed data were reviewed for quality. At the first level, statistical analysis was carried out using a general linear model approach. Contrast images were then used in fixed-effects group analyses, calculating statistically significant increases or decreases in blood oxygenation level-dependent (BOLD) signal in response to the stimuli. Group images were thresholded using cluster detection statistics, with a height threshold of $z > 2.3$ and a cluster probability of $p < .05$, corrected for whole-brain multiple comparisons using Gaussian Random Field Theory (GRFT).

2.4. Procedure

Prior to participating in the study, participants were screened over the phone to ensure that they were eligible to safely participate and met study criteria. All the remaining procedures occurred at the appointment at the Imaging Research Center at The University of Texas at Austin. Participants gave their informed consent and filled out standard MRI safety questionnaires. Then, participants completed a practice task that was similar to the task completed in the scanner but that did not focus on their rejection experience or emotional content. Participants then answered several questions relevant to their rejection experience including how resolved they currently felt about their experience on a scale from 1 (not resolved) to 7 (very resolved), how often they had thought about the situation in the past week, and how emotional, sad, hurt, angry, and rejected they felt on a scale from 1 (not at all) to 7 (very much). Participants then wrote about their rejection experience for 15-20 minutes so that the experience was salient when they began the fMRI task. During the scan, structural MRI data were acquired during the initial 5-10 minutes; then participants completed two 7-minute runs as described above. After the scan, participants were debriefed and paid for participation.

3. Results

3.1. Brain Imaging Findings

To test our hypotheses that big picture reappraisal (BPR) engages brain regions involved in cognitive control and abstraction (dlPFC, inferior and superior parietal lobe and cerebellum) BPR was compared to both rumination (see Figure 1) and distraction (see Figure 2).

Additionally, to test the hypothesis that BPR involves greater self-referential thinking than distraction (mPFC) we compared activation between the BPR and distraction conditions.

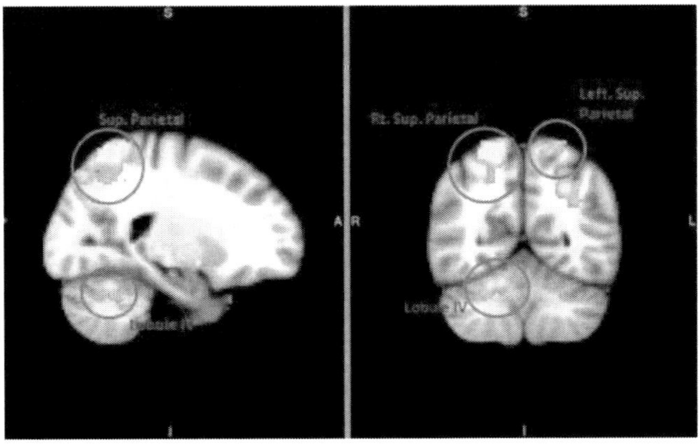

BPR>Rumination

Activation: Right Cerebellum Lobule VI. Left Superior Parietal Lobe. Sagittal View (Left) and Coronal View (Right) (Clusters 2, 3, and 4 in Table)

Figure 1. Big Picture Reappraisal (BPR)>Rumination (Rum). There was significant activation in Right Lobule VI of the Cerebellum and Right Superior Parietal activation. Rum>BPR did not yield significant activation.

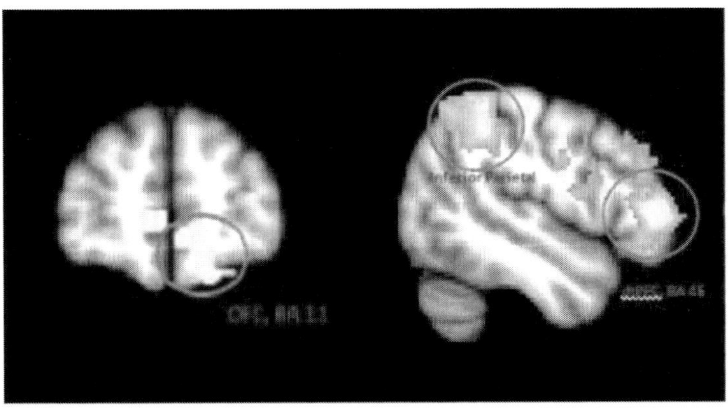

BPR versus Distraction

BPR>Dist. Left BA11(Cluster 1; Left Image) Dist>BPR. Inferior Parietal and Left BA 45,46 (Cluster 5,6; Right Image)

Figure 2. BPR>Distraction (Dist). There was significant activation in left BA 11 (OFC) and mPFC and significant activation in left BA 45,46 (Broca's area, DLPFC) and inferior parietal lobe in the Dist>BPR contrast.

3.1.1. Big Picture Reappraisal versus Rumination

In partial support of the hypotheses, this contrast yielded significant activation in bilateral superior parietal cortex and cerebellum, specifically right cerebellum lobule VI (see Table 1). Dorsolateral prefrontal cortex was not activated.

3.1.2. Big Picture Reappraisal versus Distraction

When compared to distraction, big picture reappraisal (BPR>Dist.) was hypothesized to result in self-referential thinking (mPFC) cognitive control and abstraction (dlPFC, inferior and superior parietal lobe and cerebellum; see Figure 2). This contrast resulted in partial activation of the mPFC in the cluster; however, activation was observed to a greater extent in the left OFC, or Brodmann's area (BA) 11 (see Table 1). Other hypothesized regions of interest received minimal support. To further explore these conditions given the limited findings for the hypothesized contrast, we then contrasted distraction versus big picture reappraisal (Dist>BPR). This contrast resulted in significant activation in the left prefrontal cortex that included part of Broca's area (BA 45), dlPFC (BA 46), and left inferior parietal lobe.

Table 1. Group level BOLD results threshold at cluster-corrected *p*<0.05

Cluster	Brodmann's	X	Y	Z	Z	L/R	K	Corrected p<.05
BPR>Rum								
Cluster 2		-38	-36	+64	6.25	L	4407	
Postcentral Gyrus								
Superior Parietal Lobule								
Cluster 3		+24	-54	+62	5.88	R	1336	
Superior Parietal Lobule								
Superior Lateral Occipital Cortex								
Cluster 4		+22	-58	-24	4.09	R	1133	
Cerebellum Lobule VI								
Cerebellum Lobule V								
BPR>Distract								
Cluster 1	**BA11**	-22	+60	-20	4.5	L	1310	
Orbital Frontal Cortex								
Medial Prefrontal Cortex								
Distract>BPR								
Cluster 5	**BA 45,46**	-48	+40	+6	6.03	L	2220	
Frontal Pole								
pars triangularis								
Cluster 6		-52	-42	+44	5.54	L	1838	
Inferior Parietal Lobe								
Rum>BPR		NS						

Significant clusters surrounding peak MNI (x, y, z) coordinates are listed as well as cluster Z-values. All reported values reached cluster extent threshold corrected significance of $p<0.05$. K values correspond to spatial extent (i.e., number voxels) and L/R indicate laterality of findings. (BPR=Big Picture Reappraisal, Dist=Distraction, Rum=Rumination) NS=not significant.

3.1.3. Big Picture Reappraisal versus Counting

To further test our hypothesis that big picture reappraisal (BPR) engages brain regions involved in cognitive control (inferior parietal, cerebellum, and dlPFC), self-referential thinking (mPFC) and abstraction (superior parietal), big picture reappraisal was contrasted with a counting backwards condition (see Table 2). The findings did not support the hypothesis regarding parietal activation; however.

Significant activation was found in inferior lateral occipital cortex, occipital pole, occipital fusiform gyrus, and superior lateral occipital cortex. Though unexpected, these regions may have been active in this contrast due to the visual imagery evoked when picturing an autobiographical memory compared to mental arithmetic.

Table 2. Group level BOLD results threshold at cluster-corrected

Cluster	X	Y	Z	Z	L/R	K	
							Corrected p<.05
BPR>Count							
Cluster	+32	-88	-2	9.0	R	60288	
Inferior Lateral Occipital Cortex							
Occipital Pole							
Occipital Fusiform Gyrus							
Superior Lateral Occipital Cortex							
							Uncorr. p<.05
BPR>Count							
Cluster	+32	-88	-2	9.02	R	59523	
Inferior Lateral Occipital Cortex							
Occipital Pole							
Cluster	+8	-52	-48	6.16	R	696	
Cerebellum Lobule IX							
Cluster	0	-14	+34	4.54	R	438	
Anterior Cingulate Gyrus							
Posterior Cingulate Gyrus							
Cluster	-30	-24	+58	3.76	L	425	
Precentral Gyrus							
Postcentral Gyrus							
Cluster	-16	-52	+70	3.23	L	71	
Superior Parietal Lobule							
Postcentral Gyrus							
Superior Lateral Occipital Cortex							
Cluster	-10	+14	+10	3.17	L	64	
Caudate							

Significant clusters surrounding peak MNI (x, y, z) coordinates are listed as well as cluster Z-values. All reported values reached cluster extent threshold corrected significance of $p<0.05$. K values correspond to spatial extent (i.e., number voxels) and L/R indicate laterality of findings. (BPR=Big Picture Reappraisal, Count=counting backwards (active) control condition). Uncorr.=uncorrected.

To further explore the network of brain regions that are engaged during big picture reappraisal versus counting, the contrast was analyzed at a more liberal, uncorrected p-value (p>.05). Though speculative, this contrast yielded activation of hypothesized regions including right-hemisphere cerebellum lobule IV and superior parietal lobule. Activation was also found in anterior and posterior cingulate gyrus, left-hemisphere precentral gyrus, and caudate.

3.2. Mood Data

As indicated above, we hypothesized that mood would be more positive during the distraction than the rumination induction. However, no specific hypotheses were posed regarding mood differences between BPR and the other two conditions because, while big picture thinking is expected to lead to better emotional resolution in the long run, these benefits are expected to unfold over time (Rude 2013); in addition, our BPR induction, like the rumination induction, involved an immediate focus on participants' distressing rejection experience.

As described above, mood was rated 10 times per run, initially following reminders to think about the rejection experience and then in sets of three after each set of condition-specific prompts. In order to follow this structure, each group of three mood ratings (following each set of condition-specific prompts within a run) was averaged to form a mood rating cluster. There were some missing mood ratings in the dataset and in these cases the average of the two mood ratings in the cluster was used to interpolate the third mood rating. In the case that there were not at least two mood ratings in the cluster, the data were not used. There were a total of nine instances in which cluster scores were based on only two mood ratings: Four participants' first cluster score, three participants' second cluster score, and two participants' third cluster score were based on only two mood ratings.

3.2.1. ANCOVA Analyses

The purpose of this analysis was to check for mood differences between conditions. As a first step, we checked for order effects by conducting an analysis that included Run (first, second), as well as Condition (BPR, Rumination, Distraction) as factors. Mood Clusters, averaged mood rating following each set of condition prompts (first, second, third) comprised the dependent variables and Mood Rating 1 (the rating that followed prompts to think about the rejection experience but preceded condition prompts) was included as a covariate in this analysis. Since no main effects or interactions involving Run were found (*ps* > .15), mood ıatings for the analysis were combined from Runs 1 and 2 within each condition and the above analysis was rerun without the Run factor. This analysis yielded a significant Mood Cluster by Condition interaction ($F(2,32)=3.955$; $p=.029$). To decompose this interaction, simple effects at each of the three mood cluster time points were tested by running one-way analyses of covariance (ANCOVAs) for the mood cluster at each time point, using Mood Rating 1 as the covariate, and following up significant effects with post hoc contrasts. For the first mood cluster, the one-way ANCOVA omnibus test approached significance [$F(2,34)=2.551$; $p=.09$] and was followed up. For this mood cluster, Distraction yielded significantly better mood than Big Picture Reappraisal [$F(1,25)=5.190$; $p=.03$] and trended towards significantly better mood than Rumination [[$F(1,20)=1.85$; $p=.19$]. Significant differences were not observed for mood clusters at time points 2 or 3 (*ps* > .34).

4. DISCUSSION

The present study investigated the neural substrates of emotion regulation when thinking about a real-life rejection experience and utilized a novel paradigm investigating big picture reappraisal in a group of women who had experienced recent distress. The purpose of the study was to determine if taking a big picture perspective on distress would activate brain regions associated with cognitive control (dlPFC, inferior parietal lobe, mPFC, and cerebellum) that have been shown to be active during reappraisal in previous studies. Further, this study built on past research by demonstrating that big picture reappraisal, which has been shown to improve well-being and reduce rumination (Rude et al., 2011), would also require a degree of abstract thinking (superior parietal lobe), making generalizations from more specific scenarios/information. To test these hypotheses, big picture reappraisal was contrasted with rumination, distraction because they are commonly used emotion regulation strategies and can lead to ineffective coping long term (Morrow and Nolen-Hoeksema, 1990; Nolen-Hoeksema, Wisco, and Lyubomirsky, 2008), as well as an active control.

Results, though mixed, demonstrated that big picture reappraisal engaged hypothesized brain regions including the bilateral superior parietal lobe, cerebellum, and mPFC which are involved in aspects of cognitive control, self-referential thinking, and abstraction (Koenigs et al., 2009; Ochsner et al.,

2012; Stoodley and Schmahmnn, 2009) when compared to conditions as well as an active control. However, hypothesized activation in dlPFC was not significantly greater in big picture reappraisal compared to conditions or active control. Taken together, these findings are promising and provide new information about brain activation elicited from big picture reappraisal using an ecologically valid reappraisal paradigm.

Though big picture reappraisal (when compared to distraction statements) activated a small area of a hypothesized region mPFC, the cluster extended into left OFC (BA 10) which is implicated in attributing value and valence to stimuli and regulating/attenuating arousal (Ochsner et al., 2012). The finding that distraction (compared to big picture reappraisal) resulted in activation of left dlPFC suggests that distraction also involves some aspects of cognitive control, possibility due to shifting attention away from thinking about the rejection experience to creating a mental image (Hare, Camerer, and Rangel, 2009). Together, these results suggest that there are distinct brain regions associated with implementing the cognitive coping strategies of big picture reappraisal and distraction.

In addition, compared to an active control, big picture reappraisal was hypothesized to result in bilateral superior parietal, as well as dlPFC, mPFC, and cerebellar activation. This hypothesis was not supported at the cluster-corrected $p<.05$ threshold. Activation was found in right hemisphere occipital lobe, which is involved in visual processing. This finding may be attributable, in part, to participants visualizing alternative scenarios for their rejection experience. In addition, the right hemisphere is implicated in processing emotional information (e.g., Craig, 2005), which is likely activated by one's rejection experience.

To further explore this hypothesis, the contrast was analyzed at a more liberal threshold. Though speculative, this contrast yielded activation of hypothesized regions including cerebellum and superior parietal lobe as well as right-hemisphere anterior and posterior cingulate gyrus and caudate. These findings support the hypothesis that thinking from a big picture perspective involves activation of regions associated with abstraction as well as cognitive control.

A goal of this study was to investigate the neural correlates of a specific type of reappraisal strategy which could be applied in real-life with a novel reappraisal paradigm. Left OFC, mPFC, cerebellum, and parietal lobe activation during reappraisal is consistent with previous findings for reappraisal (Ochsner et al., 2012). Importantly, big picture reappraisal compared to distraction was associated with activation of left OFC and mPFC and when compared to rumination was associated with parietal and cerebellar activation, which are areas that facilitate cognitive control of emotion and support functions such as working memory, abstraction, and valuation of stimuli. As previously mentioned, the OFC is associated with attributing value and valence to stimuli and regulating/attenuating arousal (Ochsner et al., 2012) and superior parietal cortex has been associated with abstraction and mental flexibility in previous research and those with lesions in this region can have problems with mental flexibility (Koenigs et al., 2009). In addition, right cerebellar lobule VI is associated with working memory and attention (Desmond, Gabrieli, Wagner, Ginier, and Glover, 1997; Stoodley and Schmahmann, 2009) and supports contralateral frontal regions associated with language processing and executive functioning (Allen et al., 2010; Stoodley and Schmahmann, 2009).

An important strength of the current study was its ecological validity. Only one other published study thus far has used fMRI to study reappraisal using specific appraisal instructions and using an impactful emotional stimuli from participants' lives. While prior studies that have simply asked participants to "reappraise" have contributed to our understanding, it is important to examine neural processes that accompany specific reappraisals, as was done in the present study. Further, considering an actual emotion-eliciting event, as compared to emotion-evoking pictures, is crucial toward understanding emotion regulation processes that have applicability to real-life. In addition, the study utilized a randomized design screened participants to rule out other possible factors that could have contributed to variance in brain activation beyond the treatment conditions. A limitation of the study was that the sample size was relatively small. This likely contributed to limited power to detect differences in condition contrasts at times. Finally, though using only healthy women participants reduced variability in a relatively small sample size, the generalizability of these findings to men and clinical populations is also limited.

References

Ayduk, O. and Kross, E. (2010). From a distance: implications of spontaneous self-distancing for adaptive self-reflection. *Journal of Personality and Social Psychology*, 98, 5, 809-829. doi: 10.1037/a0019205

Craig, A. D. (2005). Forebrain emotional asymmetry: a neuroanatomical basis? *Trends in Cognitive Sciences*, 9, 12, 566-571. doi:10.1016 /j.tics.2005.10.005

Desmond, J., Gabrieli, J., Wagner, A., Ginier, B., and Glover, G. (1997). Lobular patterns of cerebellar activation in verbal working-memory and finger-tapping tasks as revealed by functional MRI. *The Journal of Neuroscience*, 17, 24, 9675-9685.

Forster, K. I., and Forster, J. C. (2003). DMDX: A window display program with millisecond accuracy. *Behavior Research Methods, Instruments, and Computers*, 35, 116-124.

Gross, J. J. (2002). Emotion regulation: Affective, cognitive, and social consequences. *Psychophysiology*, 39, 281-291.

Gross, J. J., and John, O. P. (2003). Individual differences in two emotion regulation processes: Implications for affect, relationships, and well-being. *Journal of Personality and Social Psychology*, 85, 348–362.

Gyurak, A., Goodkind, M. S., Madan, A., Kramer, J. H., Miller, B. L., and Levenson, R. W. (2009). Do tests of executive functioning predict ability to downregulate emotions spontaneously and when instructed to suppress? *Cognitive, Affective, and Behavioral Neuroscience*, 9, 2, 144-152. doi: 10.3758/CABN.9.2.144

Hare, T. A., Camerer, C. F. and Rangel, A. (2009). Self-control in decision-making involves modulation of the vmPFC valuation system. *Science*, 324, 646-648. doi: 10.1126/science.1168450

Joorman, J. and Gotlib, I. H. (2010). Emotion regulation in depression: Relation to cognitive inhibition. *Cognition and Emotion*, 24, 2, 281-298. doi: 10.1080/02699930903407948

Koenigs, M., Barbey, A. K., Postle, B. R., and Grafman, J. (2009). Superior parietal cortex is crucial for the manipulation of information in working memory. *The Journal of Neuroscience*, 29, 47, 14980-14986. doi:10.1523/JNEUROSCI.3706-09.2009

Kross, E. and Ayduk, O. (2008). Facilitating adaptive emotional analysis: distinguishing distanced-analysis of depressive experiences from immersed-analysis and distraction. *Personality Social Psychology Bulletin*, 34, 924-938. doi: 10.1177/0146167208315938

Kross, E., Davidson, M., Weber, J., and Ochsner, K. (2009). Coping with emotions past: the neural basis of regulating affect associated with negative autobiographical memories. *Biological Psychiatry*. 65, 361-366. doi: 10.1016/j.biopsych.2008.10.019

Kross, E., Gard, D., Deldin, P., Clifton, J., and Ayduk, O. (2012). "Asking why" from a distance: its cognitive and emotional consequences for people with major depressive disorder, *Journal of Abnormal Psychology*, 121, 3, 559-569. doi: 10.1037/a0028808

Lantrip, C., Isquith, P., Koven, N., Welsh, K., and Roth, R. (2014, February). Relationship between Emotion Regulation Strategies and Executive Functions in Adolescents' Daily Lives. International Neuropsychological Society, Seattle, Washington.

Morrow, J., and Nolen-Hoeksema, S. (1990). Effects of responses to depression on the remediation of depressive affect. *Journal of Personality and Social Psychology*, 58, 519–527. doi: 10.1037/0022-3514.58.3.519

Nolen-Hoeksema, S., Wisco, B. E., and Lyubomirsky, S. (2008). Rethinking Rumination. *Perspectives on Psychological Science*, 3, 400-424. doi: 10.1111/j.1745-6924.2008.00088.x

Ochsner, K. N., and Gross, J. J. (2008). Cognitive emotion regulation: Insights from social cognitive and affective neuroscience. *Current Directions in Psychological Science*, 17, 153-158. doi: 10.1111/j.1467-8721.2008 .00566.x

Ochsner, K. N., Silvers, J., and Buhle, J. (2012). Functional imaging studies of emotion regulation: a synthetic review and evolving model of the cognitive control of emotion. *Annals of the New York Academy of Sciences*. 1251, E1-E24. doi: 10.1111/j.1749-6632.2012.06751.x

Olsson, A. and Ochsner, K. N. (2008). The role of social cognition in emotion. *Trends in Cognitive Sciences*, 12, 2, 65-71. doi: 10.1016/j.tics.2007 .11.010.

Ray, R., Ochsner, K., Cooper, J., Robertson, E., Gabrieli, J., and Gross, J. (2005). Individual differences in trait rumination and the neural systems supporting cognitive reappraisal. *Cognitive, Affective, and Behavioral Neuroscience,* 5, 2, 156-168.

Richards, J. and Gross, J. (2000). Emotion regulation and memory: The cognitive costs of keeping one's cool. *Journal of Personality and Social Psychology,* 79, 3, 410-424. doi: 10.1037/0022-3514.79.3.410

Rude, S.S. Miller, J., Haner, M., Gill, S., Zelmanova, J. Bruehlman-Senecal, E. (2013, May). Emotion regulation: Exploring the benefits of "big picture" appraisal. In S.S. Rude (Chair). *Symposium conducted at the meeting of the Association for Psychological Sciences*, Washington D.C.

Rude, S., Mazzetti, F., Pal, H., and Stauble, S. (2011). Social rejection: How best to think about it? *Cognitive Therapy Research.* 35, 209-216. doi: 10.1037/a0028808

Schartau, P. E., Dalgleish, T., and Dunn, B. D. (2009). Seeing the bigger picture: Training in perspective broadening reduces self-reported affect and psychophysiological response to distressing films and autobiographical memories, *Journal of Abnormal Psychology*, 118, 1, 15-27.

Schmahmann, J. D. and Sherman, J. C. (1998). The cerebellar cognitive affective syndrome, Brain, 121, 4, 561-579. doi: 10.1093/brain/121.4.561

Stoodley, C. J., and Schmahmann, J. D. (2009). Functional topography in the human cerebellum: A meta-analysis of neuroimaging studies. *Neuroimage*, 44(2), 489-501. doi: 10.1016/j.neuroimage.2008.08.039

Thompson-Schill, S. L., Bedney, M., and Goldberg, R.F. (2005). The frontal lobes and the regulation of mental activity. *Current Opinion in Neurobiology*, 15, 219-224. doi: 10.1016/j.conb.2005.03.006

In: Research Trends in Behavior …
Editor: Miao-Kun Sun

ISBN: 978-1-63485-461-0

Chapter 6

Cognitive Functioning, Decision Making and Prefrontal Cortex Damage: Consequences, Rehabilitation and Neural Plasticity

Ana Luiza Vidal Milioni[1,2], Priscila Aparecida Rodrigues[1] and Paulo Jannuzzi Cunha[2,3,4*]

[1]Institute of Physical Medicine and Rehabilitation (IMREA), Clinics Hospital, School of Medicine, University of São Paulo, Brazil
[2]Laboratory of Psychiatric Neuroimaging (LIM-21)/ Center for Interdisciplinary Research on Applied Neurosciences (NAPNA), School of Medicine, University of São Paulo, Brazil
[3]Interdisciplinary Group on Studies of Alcohol and Drugs (GREA), Institute of Psychiatry, University of São Paulo, Brazil
[4]Equilibrium Program, Institute of Psychiatry, University of São Paulo, Brazil

* Correspondence and requests for reprints: Paulo Jannuzzi Cunha, Ph.D., Laboratory of Psychiatric Neuroimaging (LIM-21)/ Center for Interdisciplinary Research on Applied Neurosciences (NAPNA), School of Medicine, University of São Paulo, Brazil. Email: pjcunha@usp.br

ABSTRACT

Traumatic brain injury (TBI) is a major problem of public health around the world. TBI is a neurological disorder that results in temporary or permanent changes in motor, cognitive and behavioral areas. It is one of the most common kinds of brain injuries in childhood/adolescence, a period in which the prefrontal cortex is in a developing process. The aim of this article is to review the neuropsychological consequences of TBI in the prefrontal cortex, as well as the valid strategies to be adopted that might contribute to a shorter recovery time of the patients. The TBI in the prefrontal cortex does not necessarily involve motor or sensorial deficits. However, it may cause functional, decision making, and social and academic impairments. More than a half of these patients develop a psychiatric disorder with disinhibiting symptoms and inappropriate behavior. Motivational, emotional, attention, perceptive and cognitive functions are mediated by the connections between the prefrontal cortex and the motor areas, the limbic system, the reticular system and the posterior association cortex. Generally, patients with TBI will present cognitive deficits associated with executive functions, decision making, problem-solving skills, judgment, and impulse control. The consequences of brain injury depend on a variety of factors, such as: the type of brain injury, intensity of the damage, extension, localization, environmental factors, age in which the TBI occurs, premorbid intelligence/cognitive reserve, and stage of cognitive development. For example, dorsolateral lesions have been associated with perseverative behavior, lack of initiative, deficit in ability to sustain and shift attention between stimuli or concepts, problem solving and working memory ("cold" executive functions). It is commonly confused with unmotivated behavior. On the other hand, ventromedial injuries have been associated with conducts based on emotional and social variables, such as inability to respond appropriately to social cues, failure to obey conventional social rules, inhibitory deficits, impulsivity and impaired decision making ("hot" executive functions). Right after the brain injury, new mechanisms of repair and reorganization of the Central Nervous System (CNS) emerge for an indefinite time period, aiming to reduce and compensate the functional impairment associated with the problem. A new neuronal circuit in the neighbor areas of the brain is established to recover lost functions and consequently to help the accomplishment of activities. The process of restructuring the brain and strengthening the cognitive functions is called neural plasticity and it can improve the prognostic of the subject at any stage of development or adult life. In most patients, when the brain injury in the prefrontal cortex happens, special educational needs or changes in the educational environment are necessary. In the meantime, there are promising treatments with stimulant drugs, neuropsychological rehabilitation, and cognitive behavioral therapy strategies. Further studies on neuropsychological rehabilitation are required to define to what extent individuals affected by TBI may have a restoration of premorbid cognitive abilities by making use of these integrated techniques.

Keywords: prefrontal cortex, executive functions, decision-making and neurodevelopment

1. Introduction

Traumatic brain injury (TBI) is a major problem of public health around the world since it is the first cause of death among children and adolescents in most of the developed countries (Arciniegas, Anderson, Topkoff and McAllister, 2005). In the United States, an estimated 1.4 million people sustain a TBI annually (Dikmen, et al., 2009). Official Reports suggest that 170 in 100,000 children will suffer TBI in the USA each year (Anderson, Godfrey, Rosenfeld and Catroppa, 2012), resulting in temporary or permanent changes in motor, cognitive and behavioral areas. TBI is one of the most common kinds of brain injuries in childhood/adolescence, a period in which the prefrontal cortex is in a developing process. The two main causes of TBI during childhood/adolescence are traffic accidents and falls. The majority of TBI in children/adolescents are mild, typically with few long-term consequences, however, a significant number of these people will suffer more serious damages and will experience physical, cognitive, educational, functional, emotional and social impairments (Stacin et al., 2002).

The brain areas work together and each part is responsible for one or more specific functions that contribute to more complex cognitive processes. For this reason, an injury in a single area of the brain may affect many functions. Considering this network of complex connections, it is hard to establish a rigid association between a specific region of the brain and a single cognitive function. Also, especially with children/adolescents, who are still acquiring new skills and brain maturity, the consequences of such damage are much more complex.

The aim of this chapter is to review the neuropsychological consequences of TBI in the prefrontal cortex, as well as the valid strategies to be adopted that might contribute to a shorter recovery time of the patients.

2. TBI: Definition and Classification

TBI is a nondegenerative and noncongenital neurological disorder that occurs after an insult to the brain caused by an external mechanical force (Ewing-Cobbs and Bloom, 1999; Koehler, Wilhelm and Shoulson, 2011).

TBI is classified as mild, moderate and severe based upon the alteration of consciousness that follows the injury. The most commonly used scale to measure the level of severity of TBI is the Glasgow Coma Scale. It has a configuration for adults and older children (Table 1) and a different one for nonverbal children, the Pediatric Glasgow Coma Scale for Nonverbal Children (Table 2). Both scales follow the same score classification: severe TBI is defined as a Glasgow Coma Scale score between 3 and 8, moderate TBI is between 9 and 12 and mild TBI is between 13 and 15.

Table 1. Glasgow Coma Scale

Behavior	Response	Score
Eye opening response	Spontaneously	4
	To speech	3
	To pain	2
	No response	1
Best verbal response	Oriented to time, place and person	5
	Confused	4
	Inappropriate words	3
	Imcomprehensible sounds	2
	No response	1
Best motor response	Obeys commands	6
	Moves to localized pain	5
	Flexion withdrawal from pain	4
	Abnormal flexoin (decorticate)	3
	Abnormal extension (decerebrate)	2
	No response	1

Behavior	Response	Score
Total score	Best response	15
	Comatose client	8 or less
	Totally unresponsive	3

There are two main types of TBI: open or closed. The Open-Type TBI occurs when an object penetrates the skull or when the skull is broken, like in wounds caused by fire guns or falls with bone perforation (Ewing-Cobbs and Bloom, 1999). In addition to physically damaging the brain, open head injuries are more likely to get an infection, which may complicate the condition. The closed-type TBI occurs when the brain collides with the inside of the skull after a crash. Even though sometimes there are no visible signals of injury, the brain can swell inside the skull, pressuring delicate neighbor tissues. In this case, there are no damages to the bone structure. It generally occurs after falls, car accidents, electric shocks and others (Dikmen et al., 2009).

Table 2. Pediatric Glasgow Coma Scale for Nonverbal Children

Behavior	Response	Score
Eye opening	Spontaneous	4
	To speech	3
	To pain	2
	No response	1
Verbal Response	Coos, babbles	5
	Irritable cry	4
	Cryng to pain	3
	Moans to pain	2
	No response	1
Motor Response	Follows commands	6
	Localizes pain	5
	Withdraws to pain	4
	Decorticate flexion	3
	Decerebrate extension	2
	No response	1

Both types of TBI frequently produce prefrontal lesions and disconnect this area from associated cortical and subcortical areas.

3. Neurodevelopment

The maturation of a child´s brain is a complex process, in which the brain grows and produces several behavioral changes, in order to adapt to the surrounding world (Aamodt and Wang, 2011). The brain of a newborn baby has higher synaptic density than the adult brain (García-Molina, Ensenat-Cantallops, Tirapu-Ustarroz and Roig-Rovira, 2009). After birth, however, the synapses form rapidly in all areas of the brain (Johnson, 2001). At the age of 3, the synaptic density reaches its peak at levels 50% higher than those found in adults (Bruer, 1998). However, it is important to remember that the peak density of synapses occur at different ages in different areas (Johnson, 2001). In this period, synaptic production outpaces the synaptic elimination and the majority of synapses are formed. This process of synaptogenesis is followed by a posterior period of synaptic pruning, in which both the environment and personal experiences play important roles (Blackmore, 2011).

4. Executive Functions

Luria (1973) proposes that the cognitive functions and the mental processes are organized in systems that embrace specific brain areas. Each of these areas (in a constant interaction with the others) plays a role in the functional system. According to the author's theory, there are 3 functional units in the brain. The first one is the arousal-motivation unit and refers to the limbic and reticular systems. The second unit is related with receiving, processing and storing information and encompasses the temporal, parietal and occipital lobes. Finally, the third unit is in charge of programming, controlling and verifying mental activity and is located in the frontal lobe (Chan, Shum, Toulopoulou and Chen, 2008). Within the frontal lobe, the prefrontal cortex is considered by Luria as the regulator of mental activity and behavior, a structure that organizes intellectual activity, programs the act and checks its performance (Luria, 1973). By this perception, the author conceptualized what is presently referred as executive functions.

Executive functions are high-level cognitive abilities that control and regulate other abilities and behaviors. They can be divided in two categories: “hot” and “cold” executive functions. The “hot” executive functions involve emotionally and motivationally influenced decisions and include the abilities of self-regulation, emotional control and theory of mind. The ventromedial and the orbitofrontal areas are responsible for the "hot" executive functions. The "cold" executive functions, on the other hand, are localized in the dorsolateral and frontostriatal areas and consist of purely cognitive abilities, such as problem-solving, mental flexibility, inhibitory control, attention and working memory (Fonseca et al., 2012).

The development of cognitive functions along the childhood and adolescence makes the subject able to process information, regulate actions and make behavior adjustments according to feedbacks from the environment. According to recent studies, the development of the executive functions begins early in life. At the age of 8 months the baby already reminds simple representations (Reznick, Morrow, Goldman and Snyder, 2004). At this age, when the baby is playing with a toy and someone hides it, he will seek for the object. During the first year of life the skill of inhibition, another kind of executive function, emerges (García-Molina et al., 2009). It can be exemplified by the fact that children at this age have the ability to interrupt a pleasure activity to attend the demand of an adult.

The development of the executive functions is connected to the maturation of the prefrontal cortex (García-Molina et al., 2009; Reznick, Morrow, Goldman and Snyder, 2004; Gogtay et al., 2004). The prefrontal grey matter has its volume increased until the age of 11 in boys and 12 in girls (Blakemore, 2010). The age difference between genders may be explained by an interaction involving puberty hormones and the grey matter development. After that, the grey matter density starts to decrease (Figure 1), reflecting the neural pruning process, a neurological regulatory process by which certain neurons and synapses are removed, leaving only efficient synaptic configuration.

Imaging studies found regional nonlinear changes in grey matter during childhood and adolescence (Gogtay et al., 2004). On the other hand, the prefrontal white matter remains on developing process during the entire childhood and adolescence, ceasing only in the second decade of life. The growth is associated to the myelination in the cortico-subcortical pathways that are associated with this brain area. It is higher in the prefrontal dorsolateral area and smaller in the prefrontal orbitofrontal regions (García-Molina et al., 2009).

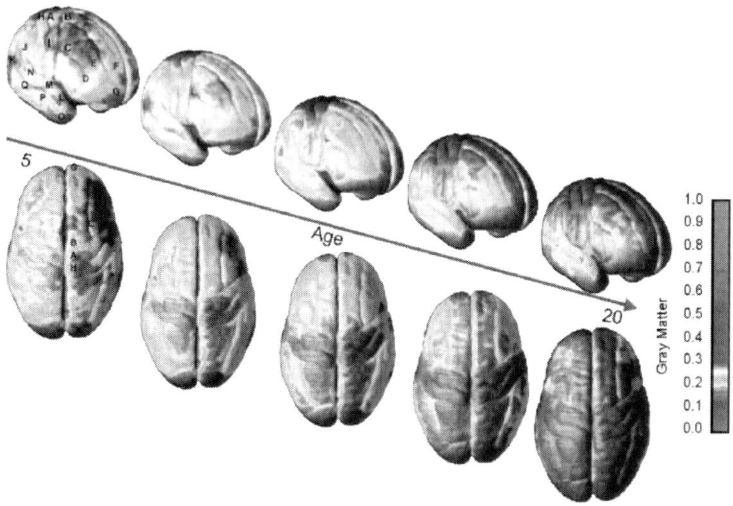

Figure 1. Right lateral and top views of the density decrease on the grey matter´s volume over the cortical surface along the maturation process (Gogtay et al., 2004).

5. Prefrontal Cortex

The prefrontal cortex seems to play a major role in the multisynaptic integration of emotion, action and experience. The entire prefrontal cortex participates in this process, but the paralimbic components have closer connection with emotion and aspects of visceral functions. The lateral part of orbitofrontal cortex (figure 2 FOC) seems to be more closely related to sensitivity to punishment whereas its medial part seems more closely related to reward (Schore, 2009).

The dorsolateral prefrontal cortex (Figure 2 F1 + F2), together with other connected areas, is especially involved with the traditional executive functions: working memory, planning ability and problem-solving (Johnson, 2001). Finally, the ventral prefrontal cortex (Fig. 2 FMC + F3t + F3o) is connected with brain regions related to emotional processing and it is responsible for behavior regulation (Johnson, 2001).

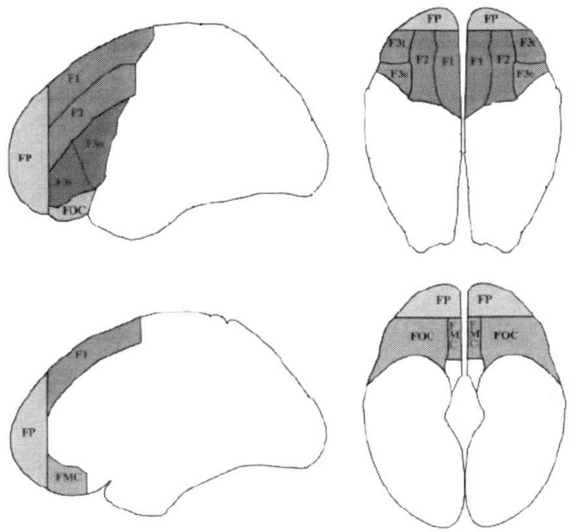

Figure 2. Parcellation units comprising the prefrontal cortical (PFC) regions of interest: frontal pole (FP; orange), dorsolateral PFC (F1 + F2; green), ventrolateral PFC (F3t + F3o; pink), ventromedial PFC (FMC; blue), orbital PFC (FOC; grey).

6. TBI and Neurodevelopment

The sequelae of TBI may include impairments in language, motor skills, processing speed, attention, learning, memory, social functions and behavioral control. These deficits may restrict the subject's ability to manage activities of daily life appropriate to life stage. For example, education and employment in the future (Anderson, Brown and Newitt, 2010; Fay et al., 1994).

In the past, it was argued that the prognosis after TBI was better in the immature brain because of the neural plasticity. This idea was initially proposed by Margaret Kenard in 1936, when studying primates (Cicchetti and Curtis, 2006). It was found that motor impairments after unilateral motor cortex injury had better prognosis in infant than in adult monkeys. This theory was generalized to humans in claiming that children would sustain less impairment and have a better recover after brain injury than adults (Dennis, 2010). The theory was named "Kenard Principle". However, in 1980 decade, studies pointed that despite the fact that the former concept is right, there are more factors to consider before taking a conclusion (Anderson et al., 1997; Kolb, Gibb and Gorny, 2000).

From a cognitive perspective, the younger the age at injury, the less consolidated are the abilities of the subject. Some of the cognitive skills are not yet established and future acquisition may be compromised. When it occurs, usually the damage is not very evident in the beginning of the recovery process and the impairments emerge with time, when the children/adolescents start showing poor or delayed skills acquisition and discrepancies among people of their age (Forsyth and Kirkham, 2012). For example, preadolescents with TBI usually have less improvement in writing than other adolescents who had TBI at an older age since the second group had already established the ability whereas the first one was still acquiring it. Studies have suggested that recovery in motor and visual-spatial functions is slower in younger adolescents than in older ones for the same reason (Thompson et al., 1994). Acquiring developmental abilities over the injury is always a challenge to the brain, which has to adapt its functioning in diverse forms (Anderson et al., 1997).

Since that the prefrontal cortex area is one of the last to become mature during the neurodevelopment, children/adolescents who had a brain injury in this region do not have all functions connected to this area established yet. For this reason, the maturation of the executive functions, the prime function of the prefrontal cortex, may have unexpected outcomes.

7. TBI in Prefrontal Cortex

Prefrontal cortex damage usually has little overt effects: the person can still walk, perceive and the cognitive impairments are not always evident in short conversations. However, it may cause many cognitive impairments, such as: deficit in attention, memory (Voytek and Knight, 2010; Tsuchida and Fellows, 2009), and decision-making processes, excessive behavioral rigidity and perseveration, a lack of empathy and inhibitory control, inappropriate social behavior (Lovell and Franzen, 1994). Interpersonal skills, judgment, socially appropriated behavior and moral conduct are related to the ability to transcend an egocentric point of view and to regulate behaviors according to the feelings and reactions of others. The impairments on this ability are particularly pronounced if prefrontal damage is acquired early in life or centered in orbitofrontal cortex (Fig. 2 FOC).

Brain injury in orbitofrontal area (Fig. 2 FOC) also presents a lack of self-control, emotional outbursts and generalized disinhibition, deficits in selective attention and problem-solving (Schore, 2009).

Patients with damage in the ventromedial (Fig. 2 FMC) components of prefrontal cortex usually prefer short-term gains in tasks in which the best strategy would be based on delayed gratifications. The absence of planning and impaired decision-making in these patients is associated with a perseverative impulse to seek immediate gratification. Dorsolateral damage (Fig. 2 F1 + F2), is related to impaired ability to shift conceptual sets, excessive behavioral rigidity and perseveration. Prefrontal cortex damage is associated with the term "dysexecutive syndrome" because it is characterized by impairments in several cognitive subdomains involving executive functions, as explained before. However, dysexecutive syndrome may be more characterized by specific alterations, depending on the specific brain region affected.

Anderson, Jacobs and Anderson (2010) suggest a list of tests to evaluate the executive functions in children/adolescents:

Attentional Control: Matching Familiar Figures (MFF; Kagan, 1966), Contingency Naming Test (CNT; Anderson et al. 2000), Trail Making Test (A-TM; Reitan, 1971), and Logan Stop Signal Task (SST; Logan 1994);

Goal Setting: Rey-Osterrieth Complex Figure (ROCFT; Rey, 1941), and Tower of London (TOL; Shallice, 1982);

Cognitive Flexibility: Controlled Oral Word Association Test (COWAT; Gaddes and Crockett, 1975, Contingency Naming Test (CNT: 3&4; Anderson et al., 2000), Concept Generation Test (CGT; Jacobs et al., 2001), Wisconsin Card Sorting Test (WCST; Heaton, 1981), and Stroop Color Word Test (SCWT; Golden, 1978); and

Executive Batteries: NEPSY (Korkman et al., 1998), BADS-C (Emslie, Wilson, Burden, Nimmo-Smith and Wilson, 2003), Preschool EF Battery (PEFB; Espy, Kaufmann, Glisky and McDiarmid, 2001), and NASAC (Anderson et al., 1995).

The use of the Frontal Assessment Battery – FAB is indicated for a screening evaluation of executive functions (Dubois et al., 2000; Cunha et al., 2010). To assess decision-making, the best instrument is the Iowa Gambling Task (IGT) (Bechara et al., 1994; Cunha et al., 2011).

8. Psychiatric Symptoms Related to TBI in Prefrontal Cortex

Since the prefrontal cortex, among its many functions, also regulates the behavior, TBI in this area leads to the development of psychiatric symptoms. According to Fay et al. (2012), 36% of the patients who had moderated or severe TBI tend to present symptoms compatible to some kinds of psychiatric disorder in the 2 years following the injury.

According to McKinlay (2002), TBI in children is associated with persisting negative effects on psychosocial development in adolescence. The study pointed out that these children were more likely to develop attention-deficit-hyperactivity disorder (ADHD), conduct disorder, substance abuse, and mood disorder. Another study (Andrews, Rose and Johnson, 1998) showed that children who had TBI presented lower self-esteem, were lonelier and had higher rates of antisocial behavior. Children who had more severe injuries showed more school problems, were engaged in fewer social activities and reported having fewer friends than the ones with less severe injury (Janusz, Kirkwood, Yeates and Taylor, 2002; Fletcher, Ewing-Cobbs, Miner, Levin and Eisenberg, 1990).

8.1. Mood Disorders: Depression, Mania, Apathy and Emotional Liability

Depression is the most common psychiatric disorder after TBI. Patients with left anterior (frontal) lesions are more likely to have depressive symptoms. The majority of patients who develop depressed mood following TBI have pre-injury risk factors, such as personal history of depressed mood or parents with a history of mood disorders (Kreutzer, Seel and Gourley, 2001). Still, depressed mood was found in subjects with no premorbid history of depression. It has also been found that TBI may increase the risk of depression, particularly in socially disadvantaged people (Kreutzer, Seel and Gourley, 2001; Vaishnavi, Rao and Fann, 2009).

Research studies suggest an incidence of mania following TBI. Van Reekum, Cohen and Wong (2000) revised several studies and found that 4.2% of all subjects who had the diagnosis of mania were directly caused by TBI. Mania disorder following TBI usually presents more aggressive and irritable symptoms and less euphoria. Predisposing factors for development of mania after TBI are damage to the basal region of right temporal lobe and right orbitofrontal cortex and individuals with family history of bipolar disorder (Mustafa, Evrim and Sarı, 2005).

Also, Max et al. (2000) used the Neuropsychiatric Rating Scale in 94 children and adolescents with ages between 5 and 14 and found mood liability in 49% of the subjects and apathy in 14%.

8.2. Anxiety

Overanxious disorders, specific phobias, separation anxiety disorders, and social anxiety disorders reflect the various types of anxiety that patients often experience following brain injury. TBI, especially with prefrontal cortex damage, is associated with an increased incidence of anxiety symptoms. The amygdala is central to the development and expression of conditioned fear reactions, and studies in humans and animals have shown that learning to inhibit these fear reactions involves inhibition by the ventral medial prefrontal cortex (Etkin, Egner and Kalisch, 2011). Patients with anxiety symptoms have diminished activation of the ventral medial prefrontal cortex during the processing of fear. It is possible that a person's capacity to regulate the fear reaction may be impaired after mild TBI, because the neural networks involved in the regulation of anxiety may be damaged as a result of the TBI (Byrant, 2008; 2011; Simmons and Matthews, 2012). TBI also decreases the neurotrophic factor levels such as vascular endothelial growth factor (VEGF) in the PFC which is known as anxiolytic. The change in VEGF levels alters the cell proliferation and maturation in the brain region such as PFC (Baykara et al., 2012).

8.3. Substance Abuse, Gambling and Other Compulsive Behavior

Investigations suggest that prefrontal cortex dysfunction may produce impulsive behavior and greater risk for substance use disorders (Chambers, Taylor and Potenza, 2003). There are also evidences that TBI may increase drug or alcohol use in persons with no histories of significant substance use prior to the injury, especially if the injury reaches the orbitofrontal cortex (Bjork and Grant, 2009).

Since TBI in the prefrontal cortex has a great impact on executive functions, increased preference for small-immediate rewards over large-delayed rewards is expected (McHugh and Wood, 2008). In a betting game, subjects who had TBI also made more impulsive choices, and responded suboptimally to changes in reward probability (Salmond and Jacquelyn, 2005). This happens because of the disability in the regulation of motivational behavior, recompenses systems and inhibitory control. This preference for immediate recompense is also observable in individuals addicted to substances, which suggests that people who had TBI, especially those with prefrontal injury, may be impaired in their ability to generate a mental representation of potential long-term negative consequences of drug use, a process also called "Miopia for the Future" (Bjork and Grant, 2009; Bechara et al., 1994). The problem is even worse in substance dependents with previous symptoms of inattention and impulsivity (Cunha et al, 2013).

8.4. Psychosis

Psychosis secondary to TBI is reported to occur in anywhere from 4% to 8.9% of individuals who sustained TBI (Fujii, 2002). McAllister and Ferrell (2000) have noted a connection between the development of psychotic symptoms and orbital frontal, temporal, and basal ganglia damage following TBI. Although there are evidences that TBI in the prefrontal cortex and psychosis are connected, the significance of this association has not been clarified yet.

8.5. Conduct Disorder and Aggressive Behavior

Studies suggest that lesions to the prefrontal cortex early in life are strictly connected to the development of antisocial and aggressive behavior in children and adolescents (Raine, 2002). Pennington and Bennetto (1993) investigated nine cases of children who had frontal lesions in the first 10 years of life. All of the subjects developed behavioral problems, 7 of them having conduct disorder.

9. TBI and Prognostic Predictors

Cognitive reserve and environmental factors are also predictors of the long-term prognosis. Cognitive reserve is a concept that was developed to explain inter-individual variability in the response to brain damage and neurological disorders. Higher preinjury cognitive reserve has been linked to a higher level of intellectual functioning after the injury. Definitions of cognitive reserve have generally used preinjury intellectual level (IQ) to be determined. According to Kirkwood, Yeates, Randolph and Kirk (2012), there are many tests which may evaluate the premorbid IQ of the children/adolescents who had a TBI. The Wechsler Intelligence Scale for Children – Fourth Edition (WISC–IV), is one of the most utilized instruments to evaluate intelligence thought diverse sub-tests, especially those used to evaluate consolidated verbal abilities such as Vocabulary and Information (Lezak et al., 2004). Even when TBI is diffuse or bilateral, Vocabulary tends to be among the least affected of the WISC battery tests (Lezak et al., 2004). Also, the California Verbal Learning Test–Children's Version (CVLT–C) measures verbal learning and memory. The Grooved Pegboard evaluates speed and dexterity of the fine motor coordination. The Woodcock–Johnson III Tests of Achievement (WJ–III) evaluates Reading ability and Word Memory Test (WMT), evocation ability, respectively. Level of education, brain size and academic achievement have all been found to be positively related to prognosis as well (Howieson, Loring and Hannay, 2004). The best outcomes have been associated to good social support and family cohesion. Genetic characteristics may also play a role in this process, but further studies are necessary to address to what extent the interaction between genetic, premorbid cognitive reserve and environmental factors are crucial for the rehabilitation process.

10. Neuroplasticity after TBI

Studies with animals suggest that the neurochemical environment of the brain after TBI (as well as others brain injuries) becomes more "immature" (Cramer and Chopp, 2000), which facilitates the plasticity occurrence. However, such plasticity is not always functional. The adaptive plasticity after TBI is usually the one that happens after relearning and practical action in the remaining neural network (Forsyth and Kirkham, 2012).

11. Recovery Strategies

11.1. Neuropsychological Evaluation

Neuropsychology is a specialty of the psychology which investigates the association between brain structure and neurocognitive functioning, considering the psychological processes and behaviors in both normal and abnormal conditions (Lezak et al, 2004). The neuropsychological evaluation is a method that combines investigation about the patient complain and testing. The results may guide the professional to effective treatment methods for the rehabilitation of patients by indicating which cognitive abilities are intact and which ones have been impaired and to what degrees. A careful Neuropsychological Evaluation is always a very important procedure to investigate cognitive strengthens and weaknesses after TBI, such as whether verbal or visual functions are more depressed, and the extent to which retrieval memory problems, frontal behavioral disinhibition, or impaired executive functioning, each of which might contribute to the poor performance on daily and educational tasks (Hannay, Howieson, Loring, Fischer and Lezak, 2004).

11.2. Cognitive Rehabilitation

The goal of the cognitive rehabilitation with TBI patients is to assist the individual in the process of recovering or compensating the damaged cognitive functions so he/she can move through daily life. The restorative approach is focused on reinforcing the functions that remain at least in some extent intact. The compensatory approach focuses on training the patients on new strategies to cope with the impairment (Freire, Coelho, Lacerda, 2011). The cognitive rehabilitation treatment varies, depending on individual deficits. Usually, a neuropsychological evaluation is completed to determine which and how the cognitive functions may be trained before the treatment with cognitive rehabilitation begins. The treatment involves the training of day life activities and repetitive exercises of writing, drawing and verbal processes.

11.3. Family

Successful rehabilitation requires family cooperation in a variety of areas such as transportation, finances, leisure, and emotional support (Jacobs, 1988).

Family functioning has been associated with greater improvement in people with TBI, including improvement in overall disability, level of functioning, and employability in the future. The family may be helpful by proposing activities, after they get oriented by professionals, and motivating the child/adolescent. The person with injury may be more vulnerable to environmental stressors that might make the recovery more difficult and also impede the recovery process. Caregiver distress may diminish the effectiveness of rehabilitation. Unfortunately, there is evidence that family members experience substantial emotional distress and family dysfunction after injury (Sander, Maestas, Sherer, Malec and Richardson, 2012). Parents can also stimulate patients with TBI in the PRC by encouraging them to play board games, for example. Children and adolescents must be stimulated to exercise as much self-control as possible in the context of enjoyable experiences such as playing, since this activity require them to resist impulses (Aamodt and Wang, 2011). Structured play with other people can also improve executive function, cognitive flexibility, and social interaction. A recent study combining Motivational Interviewing with chess showed improvement of working memory in addicted patients, therefore the "Motivational Chess" could be an interesting strategy to be used with patients suffering from other types of prefrontal damage (Gonçalves et al., 2014)

11.4. School

Patients who have physical impairments associated with the TBI are most easily comprehended. For example, when a child/adolescent enters the classroom in a wheelchair, for example, the teachers as well as the other students, are reminded that he has sustained injuries. On the other hand, when the subject who had TBI in prefrontal cortex seems healthy, walking and interacting with no obvious physical deficits, people tend to assume that he is completely recovered and requires no academic or behavioral assistance. Educators are usually not prepared to deal with students who had TBI. They currently have a limited behavioral repertory to assist those students once they are back to classroom (Berbaum, 2007). Unfortunately, there are no usual procedures or curricula specifically for students with TBI. According to Vygotsky (1978) and his concept of Zone of Proximal Development (ZPD), the learning process may be stimulated by an interactive environment, in which the teacher and other students may contribute to the development of cognitive abilities of the learner. The ZPD is, basically, the difference between what a learner can do alone and what he can do with help (Hedegaard, 2005). According to Shabani, Khatib and Ebadi (2010), the learner may be kept in his own ZPD as often as possible by solving tasks that are slightly harder than what he is able to do by himself. The aim of this process is that, after completing the task with help (sometimes more than once), the individual may be able to do the same thing alone. When the learner is a child/adolescent who had TBI in prefrontal cortex, the applying of this method is even more important. By working with help, the individual identifies his own potential, which motivates them in the learning process. Besides that, by the repetition, in peers, of activities that require more abilities than he has at the moment, the subjects may adapt skills and develop new ones to complete the activity.

Berbaum (2007) suggests that there are two essential forms to assist the patients who had TBI in the learning process: adaptation of the learning environment and accommodation of the student impairment. Adaptation occurs by the use of alternative strategies to evaluate the student academic skills, as well as altering the presentation mode to make the comprehension easier. Accommodation includes modification of demands and expectations for the student according to his/her abilities and competencies in specific skill domains.

Tyler, Blosser, and DePompei (1999) provided a list with common difficulties of patients who had TBI at school and suggestions about how to deal with it:

Concentration/attention: reduce distractions; divide activities in smaller units so the student can complete one section at time; and ask the student to review the information that has been presented; and create a signaling system to ask the student to pay attention;

Memory: regularly repeat and summarize information; orient the student to use devices (calendars, sticky notes, etc.) to compensate memory impairments; and link the new information with the student's relevant previous knowledge; and

Organization: provide for the student extra time to review his/her work; and checklists of steps for complex tasks.

11.5. Pharmacological Strategies

Because of the diversity of symptoms in patients with TBI and the differences in the form that any individual may react to a medication, there is no general pharmacologic treatment for people who had TBI. The individual symptoms must be carefully observed before the treatment is planned. As it has been said before, TBI in prefrontal cortex may cause neuropsychiatric symptoms, neurocognitive deficits and neurobehavioral impairments. The most commonly medication used in these cases are:

Stimulants. TBI is associated with decreased dopamine activity and stimulants increases extracellular dopamine levels, especially in the frontal cortex.

The most commonly used stimulant by people who had TBI is methylphenidate. The literature reports that it has been safely used in adults and pediatric patients with positive effects on cognitive functions including memory, executive functions, attention and global cognition (Writer and Schillerstrom, 2009; Talsky et al., 2010).

Nonstimulant dopamine enhancers (antiparkinsonian drugs). Like the simulants, these drugs serve to increase dopamine levels in the brain. They may function as an agonist or a dopamine precursor. The most commonly used types are amantadine, bromocriptine, pramipexole and carbidopa (Talsky et al., 2010). Studies reported that nonstimulant dopamine enhancers improve executive functioning, attention, global cognitive functioning, memory and language in adults and pediatric patients who had TBI (Writer and Schillerstrom, 2009).

Acetylcholinesterase Inhibitors. Acetylcholinesterase inhibitors increase the acetylcholine levels and restore regular cholinergic synaptic transmission, which is impaired by TBI. Studies (Zhang, Plotkin and Wang, 2004; Tenovuo, 2005) related that acetylcholinesterase inhibitors do have a positive impact on neurocognitive abilities of patients who had TBI, notably in memory and attention.

Mood Stabilizers (Anticonvulsants). This class of medication embraces drugs such as valproic acid, carbamazepine, lamotrigine, and oxcarbazepine. These anticonvulsants are used in the treatment of violent behaviors, bipolar symptomatology, manic symptoms, and liability of mood. They may be useful in the treatment of neuropsychiatric symptoms of TBI patients, but their impact in cognitive skills is still a controversy (Talsky et al., 2010). Smith et al. (1994) reported that long-term carbamazepine use in TBI adults and pediatric patients had negative effects on cognition including executive functioning, sensory-motor-perceptual skills, and attention. Other studies (Chatham-Showalter and Kimmel, 2000; Dikmen et al., 2000) have suggested that valproic acid have positive neurocognitive effects including improved recent memory and problem-solving abilities, but also have a negative impact on decision-making speed.

Antidepressants. Evidences suggest that antidepressant can be useful on the treatment of both neuropsychiatric and neurocognitive deficits persisting from TBI (Talsky et al., 2010). The use of selective serotonin reuptake inhibitors (SSRIs) have shown to improve behavior, neurocognitive and neuropsychiatric deficits, particularly agitation, depression, psychomotor retardation and recent memory lost (Writer and Schillerstrom, 2009).

Conclusion

The neuropsychological consequences of TBI in the prefrontal cortex are very complex and depend on a variety of factors. All the valid strategies to be adopted after TBI must include an integration of behavioral, familiar, educational and pharmacological approaches, which may contribute to a shorter recovery time of the young people in development. There are promising treatments with stimulant drugs and neuropsychological rehabilitation, but further studies are required to define to what extent individuals affected by TBI may have a complete restoration (or not) of premorbid cognitive abilities through using these integrated techniques.

Acknowledgment

Dr. Paulo Jannuzzi Cunha would like to thank FAPESP (Grant 2010/15604-0).

References

Aamodt, S. and Wang, S. (2011). *Welcome to your child's brain: How the mind grows from conception to college*. New York: Ed. Bloomsburry.

Anderson, C. V., Bigler, E. D, and Blatter, D. D. (1995). Frontal lobe lesions, diffuse damage, and neuropsychological functioning in traumatic brain-injured patients. *Journal of Clinical and Experimental Neuropsychology*, 17(6), 900-908.

Anderson, P., Anderson V., Northam, E., and Taylor, H. G. (2000). Standardization of the Contingency Naming Test for school-aged children: a new measure of reactive flexibility. *Clinical Neuropsychological Assesment,* 1, 247-273.

Anderson, V., Godfrey, C., Rosenfeld, J. V., and Catroppa, C. (2012). 10 years outcome from childhood traumatic brain injury. *International Journal of Developmental Neuroscience*, 30, 217-224.

Anderson, V. A., Brown, S., and Newitt, H. (2010). What Contributes to Quality of Life in Adult Survivors of Childhood Traumatic Brain Injury?. *Journal of Neurotrauma*, 27, 863-870.

Anderson, V. A., Morse, S.A., Klug, G., Catroppa, C., Harito,u F., Rosenfeld, J., and Pentland, L. (1997). Predicting recovery from head injury in young children: A prospective analysis. *Journal of the International Neuropsychological Society*, 3, 568-580.

Andrews, T. K., Rose, F. D., and Johnson, D. A. (1998). Social and behavioral effects of traumatic brain injury in children. *Brain Injury*, 12, 133-138.

Arciniegas, D. B., Anderson, C. A., Topkoff, J., and McAllister, T. W. (2005). Mild traumatic brain injury: a neuropsychiatric approach to diagnosis, evaluation, and treatment. *Neuropsychiatric Disease and Treatment*, 1(4), 311-327.

Baykara, B., Cetin, F., Baykara, B., Aksu, I., Dayi, A., Kiray, M., Sisman, A.R., Ozdemir, D., Arda, M.N., and Uysal, N. (2012). Anxiety Caused by Traumatic Brain Injury Correlates to Decreased Prefrontal Cortex Vegf Immunoreactivity and Neuron Density in Immature Rats. *Turkish Neurosurgery*, 22(5), 604-610.

Bechara, A., Damasio, A. R., Damasio, H., and Anderson, S. W. (1994). Insensitivity to future consequences following damage to human prefrontal cortex. *Cognition*, 50, 7-15.

Berbaum, C. (2007). School Reintegration Following Traumatic Brain Injury in Children and Adolescents. *Dissertation Abstracts International Section A: Humanities and Social Sciences*, Walden University.

Bjork, J. M. and Grant, S. J. (2009). Does Traumatic Brain Injury Increase Risk for Substance Abuse?. *Journal of Neurotrauma*, 26(7), 1077-1082.

Blackmore, S. J. (2008). Special Issue: Neurocognitive Approaches to Developmental Disorders: A Festschrift for Uta Frith. *The Quarterly Journal of Experimental Psychology*, 61(1), 40-49.

Blackmore, S. J. (2011). Imaging brain development: The adolescent brain. *Neuroimage,* 61(2), 397-406.

Blackmore, S. J., Burnett, S., and Dahl, R. E. (2010). The role of puberty in the developing adolescent brain. Human Brain Mapping, 31(6), 926-933.

Bruer, J. T. (1998). The brain and child development: time for some critical thinking. *Public Health Reports*, 113, 388-397.

Byrant, R. A. (2008). Disentangling mild traumatic brain injury and stress reactions. *Journal of Traumatic Stress*, 9(3), 621-629.

Byrant, R. A. (2011). Post-traumatic stress disorder vs traumatic brain injury. *Dialogues in Clinical Neurosciense*. 13(3), 251-262.

Chambers, R. A., Taylor, J. R., and Potenza, M. N. (2003). Developmental Neurocircuitry of Motivation in Adolescence: A Critical Period of Addiction Vulnerability. *American Journal of Psychiatry*, 160(6), 1041-1052.

Chan, R. C. K., Shum, D., Toulopoulou, T., and Chen, E. Y. H. (2008). Assessment of executive functions: Review of instruments and identification of critical issues. *Archives of Clinical Neuropsychology*, 23, 201-216.

Chatham-Showalter, P., and Kimmel, D. N. (2000) Agitated symptom response to divalproex following acute brain injury. *Journal Neuropsychiatry Clinical Neuroscience*, 12, 395-397.

Cicchetti, D. and Curtis, W. J. (2006). The Developing Brain and Neural Plasticity: Implications for Normality, Psychopathology, and Resilience. In: *Developmental Psychopathology: Developmental Neuroscience* (Vol. 2) (pp. 1-64). New York: Wiley.

Cramer, S. C., Chopp, M. (2000). Recovery recapitulates ontogeny. *Trends Neuroscience,* 23, 265-71.

Cunha, P. J., Bechara, A., de Andrade, A. G., and Nicastri, S. (2011). Decision-making deficits linked to real-life social dysfunction in crack cocaine-dependent individuals. *American Journal of Addictions*, 20, 78-86.

Cunha, P. J., Gonçalves, P. D., Ometto, M., Dos Santos, B., Nicastri, S., Busatto, G. F., and de Andrade, A. G. (2013). Executive cognitive dysfunction and ADHD in cocaine dependence: searching for a common cognitive endophenotype for addictive disorders. *Frontiers in Psychiatry*, 21, 126. doi: 10.3389/fpsyt.2013.00126. eCollection 2013.

Cunha, P. J., Nicastri, S., de Andrade, A. G., and Bolla, K. I. (2010). The frontal assessment battery (FAB) reveals neurocognitive dysfunction in substance-dependent individuals in distinct executive domains: Abstract reasoning, motor programming, and cognitive flexibility. *Addictive Behaviors,* 35, 875-81.

Dennis, M. (2010). Margaret Kennard (1899–1975): Not a 'Principle' of Brain Plasticity but a Founding Mother of Developmental Neuropsychology. *Cortex,* 46(8), 1043-1059.

Dikmen, S. Machamer, J.E., Winn, H.R., Anderson, G.D., and Temkin, N.R. (2000). Neuropsychological effects of valproate in traumatic brain injury. *Neurology,* 54, 895-902.

Dikmen, S. S. Corrigan, J.D., Levin, H.S., Machamer, J., Stiers, W., and Weisskopf, M.G. (2009). Cognitive Outcome Following Traumatic Brain Injury. *Journal of Head Trauma Rehabilitation,* 24(6), 430-438.

Dubois, B., Slachevsky, A., Litvan, I., and Pillon, B. (2000). The FAB: a Frontal Assessment Battery at bedside. *Neurology*, 55(11), 1621-1626.

Emslie H., Wilson F. C., Burden V., Nimmo-Smith I. and Wilson B. A. (2003) Behavioural Assessment of the Dysexecutive Syndrome for Children (BADS-C). Child Neuropsychology,13, 539-542.

Epsy, K. A., Kaufmann, P. M., McDiarmid, M. D., and Glisky, M. L. (2001). New procedures to access executive functions in preschool children. *The Clinical Neuropsychologist,* 15(1), 46-58.

Etkin, A., Egner, T., and Kalisch, R. Emotional processing in anterior cingulate and medial prefrontal cortex. *Trends in Cognitive Sciences*, 15(9), 85-93.

Ewing-Cobbs, L. and Bloom, D. R. (1999). Traumatic Brain Injury (pp. 262-288). In: Brown, R. T. *Cognitive aspects of chronic illness in children.* NY: The Guilford Press.

Fay, G. C., Jaffe, K. M., Polissar, N. L., Liao, S., Rivara, J. B., and Martin, K.M. (1994). Outcome of pediatric traumatic brain injury at three years: A cohort study. *Archives of Physical Medicine and Rehabilitation*, 75, 733-741.

Fay, T. B., Yeates, K. O., Wade, S. L., Drotar, D., Stancin, T., and Taylor, H. G. (2009). Predicting longitudinal patterns of functional deficits in children with traumatic brain injury. *Neuropsychology*, 23(3), 271-282.

Fletcher, J. M., Ewing-Cobbs, L., Miner, M. E., Levin, H. S., and Eisenberg, H. M. (1990). Behavioral changes after closed head injury in children. *Journal of Consulting and Clinical Psychology*, 58(1), 93-98.

Fonseca, R., Zimmermann, N., Cotrena, C., Cardoso, C., Kristensen, C. H., Grassi-and Oliveira, R. (2012). Neuropsychological assessment of executive functions in traumatic brain injury: hot and cold components. *Psychology and Neuroscience*, 5(2), 183-190.

Forsyth, R. and Kirkham, F. (2012). Predicting outcome after childhood brain injury. *Canadian Medical Association or its licensors*, 184(11), 1257-1264.

Freire, F. R., Coelho, F., Lacerda, J.R.; da Silva, M.F., Gonçalves, V.T., Machado, S., Velasques, B., Ribeiro, P., Basile, L.F.H., Oliveira, A.M.P., Wellingson Paiva, W.S., Kanda, P.A.M., and Anghinah, R. (2011). Cognitive rehabilitation following traumatic brain injury. Dementia and *Neuropsychologia,* 5(1), 17-25.

Fujii, D. (2002). Neuropsychiatry of Psychosis Secondary to Traumatic Brain Injury. *Psychiatric Times*, 19(8), 1-2.

Gaddes, W. H. and Crockett, D. J. (1975). The Spreen Benton Aphasia Tests: Normative data as a measure of normal language development. Brain and Language, 2, 257-279.

García-Molina, A., Ensenat-Cantallops, A, Tirapu-Ustarroz, J., and Roig-Rovira, T. (2009). Maduración de la corteza prefrontal y desarrollo de las funciones ejecutivas durante los primeros cinco años de vida. *Revista de Neurología,* 48(8), 435-440.

Gogtay, N., Giedd, J.N., Lusk, L., Hayashi, K.M., Greenstein, D., Vaituzis, A.C., Nugent, T.F. 3rd, Herman, D.H., Clasen, L.S., Toga, A.W., Rapoport, J.L., and Thompson, P.M. (2004). Dynamic mapping of human cortical development during childhood through early adulthood. *Proceedings of the National Academy of Sciences of the United States of America,* 101(21), 8174-8179.

Golden, C. J. (1978). *Stroop color and word test: A manual for clinical and experimental users* (pp.1-32). Chicago: Skoelting Company.

Gonçalves, P. D., Ometto, M., Bechara, A., Malbergier, A., Amaral, R., Nicastri, S., Martins, P. A., Beraldo, L., dos Santos, B., Fuentes, D., Andrade, A. G., Busatto, G. F., and Cunha, P. J. (2014). Motivational interviewing combined with chess accelerates improvement in executive functions in cocaine dependent patients: a one-month prospective study. *Drug and Alcohol Dependence*, 141, 79-84.

Hannay, H. J., Howieson, D. B., Loring, D. W., Fischer, J. S., and Lezak, M. D. (2004). Neuropathology for Neuropsychologists. In Lezak, M. D., Howieson, D. B., Loring, D. W. (Org.), *Neuropsychological Assessment* (pp. 157-285). New York: Oxford University Press.

Heaton, R. (1981). *A manual for the Wisconsin Card Sorting Test*. Florida: Psychological Assesment Resources.

Hedegaard, M. (2005). The zone of proximal development as basis for instruction (pp. 225-284). In: Daniels, H. *An introduction to Vygotsky*. USA: Ed. Routledge.

Howieson, D. B., Loring, D. W., and Hannay, H. J. (2004). Neurobehavioral Variables and Diagnostic Issues. In Lezak, M. D., Howieson, D. B., Loring, D. W. (Org.), *Neuropsychological Assessment* (pp. 286-336). New York: Oxford University Press.

Jacobs, R., Anderson, V., and Harvey, A. S. (2001). Concept Generation Test: A measure of conceptual reasoning skills in children. Examination of developmental trends. *Clinical Neuropsychological Assessment*, 2, 101-117.

Jacobs, H. E. (1988). Vocational rehabilitation (pp. 245-284). In Liberman, R. P. Psychiatn'c *Rehabilitation of Chronic Mental Patients*. Washington, DC: American Psychiatric Press.

Janusz, J. A., Kirkwood, M. W., Yeates, K. O., and Taylor, H. G. (2002). Social problem-solving skills in children with traumatic brain injury: long-term outcomes and prediction of social competence. *Child Neuropsychology,* 8, 179-194.

Johnson, M. H. (2001) Functional brain development in humans. *Nature reviews*. N*euroscience*, 2, 475-483.

Kagan, J. (1966). Reflection-impulsity: The generality and dynamics of conceptual temp. *Journal of Abnormal Psychology*, 71, 75-81.

Kalia, M. (2008). Brain development: anatomy, connectivity, adaptive plasticity, and toxicity. *Metabolism*, 57(2), S2-S5.

Kirkwood, M. W., Yeates, K. O., Randolph, C. K., and Kirk, J. W. (2012). The implications of symptom validity test failure for ability-based test performance in a pediatric sample. *Psychological Assessment*,24(1), 36-45.

Koehler, R., Wilhem, E., and Shoulson, I. (2011). Cognitive Rehabilitation Therapy for Traumatic Brain Injury: Evaluating the Evidence. Institute of Medicine of the National Academies.Washington: The National Academies Press. pp. 1-272.

Kolb, B., Gibb, R., and Gorny, G. (2000). Cortical plasticity and the development of behavior after early frontal cortical injury. *Developmental Neuropsychology,* 18, 423-44.

Korkman, M., Kirk, U., and Kemp S. (1998). NEPSY-A Developmental Neuropsychological Assessment. Texas: The Psychological Corporation.

Kreutzer, J. S., Seel, R. T., and Gourley, E. (2001). The prevalence and symptom rates of depression after traumatic brain injury: a comprehensive examination. *Brain Injury,* 15 (7), 563-576.

Lezak, M. D., Howieson, D. B., and Loring, D. W. (2004). *Neuropsychological Assessment – Fourth Edition.* New York: Oxford University Press.

Logan, G. D. (1994). On the ability to inhibit thought and action: A users guide to the stop-signal paradigm. In: Dagenbach, D., Carr, T. H. *Inhibitory processes in attention, memory, and language.* (pp. 189–239). San Diego: Academic Press.

Lovell, M. R. and Franzen, M. D. (1994). Neuropsychological Assessment. In: Silver, J. M., Yudofsky, S. C., Hales, R. E. (Org.), *Neuropsychiatry of traumatic brain injury.* (pp. 133-160). American Psychiatric Press.

Luria, A. R. (1973). *The Working brain: An introduction to neuropsychology.* New York: Basic.

Max, J. E., Robin, D.A., Lindgren, S.D., Smith, W.L. Jr, Sato, Y., Mattheis, P.J., Stierwalt, J.A., and Castillo, C.S. (1998). Traumatic Brain Injury in Children and Adolescents: Psychiatric Disorders at Two Years. *Journal of the American Academy of Child and Adolescent Psychiatry*, 36(9), 1278-1285.

Max, J. E., Koele, S.L., Castillo, C.C., Lindgren, S.D., Arndt, S., Bokura, H., Robin, D.A., Smith, W.L. Jr, and Sato, Y. (2000). Personality change disorder in children and adolescents following traumatic brain injury. *Journal of International Neuropsychological Society*, 6(3), 279-289.

McAllister, T. W. and Ferrell, R. B. (2000). Evaluation and treatment of psychosis after traumatic brain injury. *NeuroRehabilitati*on, 17, 357-368.

McHugh., L. and Wood, R. L. (2008) Using a temporal discounting paradigm to measure decision-making and impulsivity following traumatic brain injury: a pilot study. *Brain Inj*, 22, 715–721.

McKinlay, A., Grace, R. C., Horwood, L. J., Fergusson, D. M., and MacFarlane, M. R. (2010). Long-term behavioural outcomes of pre-school mild traumatic brain injury. *Child: Care, Health and Development*, 36, 22-30.

Mustafa, B., Evrim, O., and Sari, A. (2005). Secondary Mania Following Traumatic Brain Injury. *The Journal of Neuropsychiatry and Clinical Neurosciences,* 17(1), 122-124.

Pennington, B. F. and Bennetto, L. (1993). Main effects or transactions in the neuropsychology of conduct disorder? Commentary on "The neuropsychology of conduct disorder". *Development and Psychopathology,* 5, 153–164.

Raine, A. (2002). Annotation: The role of prefrontal deficits, low autonomic arousal, and early health factors in the development of antisocial and aggressive behavior in children. *Journal of Child Psychology and Psychiatry,* 43(4), 417-434.

Reitan, R. M. (1971). Trail Making Test Results for Normal and Brain-Damaged Children. *Perceptual and Motor Skills,* 33, 575-581.

Rey, A. (1941). Psychological examination of traumatic encephalopathy. Archives de Psychologie, 28, 286–340.

Reznick, J. S, Morrow, J. D., Goldman, B. D., and Snyder, J. (2004). The onset of working memory in infants. *Infancy*, 6, 145-54.

Salmond, C. H., Jacquelyn, S. B. (2005). Cognitive outcome in traumatic brain injury survivors. *Neuroscience*, 11(2), 111-116.

Sander, A. M., Maestas, K. L., Sherer, M., Malec, J. F., and Richardson, R. N. (2012). Relationship of Caregiver and Family Functioning to Participation Outcomes After Postacute Rehabilitation for Traumatic Brain Injury: A Multicenter Investigation. Archives of Physical Medicine and Rehabilitation, 93, 842-848.

Shabani, K., Khatib, M., and Ebadi, S. (2010) Vygotsky's Zone of Proximal Development: Instructional Implications and Teachers' Professional Development. *Canadian Center of Science and Education*, 3(4), 237-248.

Shallice T. (1982). Specific impairments of planning. *Philosophical Transactions of the Royal Society London*, 298, 199–209.

Smith, K.R. Jr, Goulding, P.M., Wilderman, D., Goldfader, P.R., Holterman-Hommes, P., and Wei, F. (1994). Neurobehavioral effects of phenytoin and carbamazepine in patients recovering from brain trauma: a comparative study. *Archives of Neurology*, 51, 653–660.

Simmons, A. N. and Matthews, S. C. (2012). Neural circuitry of PTSD with or without mild traumatic brain injury: A meta-analysis. *Neuropharmacology*, 62, 598-606.

Stancin, T., Drotar, D., Taylor, H.G., Yeates, K.O., Wade, S.L., and Minich, N.M. (2002). Health-Related Quality of Life of Children and Adolescents After Traumatic Brain Injury. *Pediatrics,* 109, E34

Talsky, A. et al. (2010). Pharmacological interventions for traumatic brain injury. *British Columbia Medical Journal*, 53(1), p. 1.

Tenovuo, O. (2005). Central acetylcholinesterase inhibitors in the treatment of chronic traumatic brain injury-clinical experience in 111 patients.

Progress in Neuropsychopharmacology and Biological Psychiatry, 29(1), 61-67.

Thompson, N. M., Kojima, M., and Higuchi, Y. (1994). Motor, visuo-spatial, and somatosensory skills after closed head injury in children and adolescents: A study of change. *Neuropsychology*, 8, 333–342.

Tsuchida, A. and Fellows, L. K. (2009). Lesion evidence that two distinct regions within prefrontal cortex are critical for n-back performance in humans. *Neuroscience*, 21, 2263–2275.

Tyler, J., Blosser, J., and Depompei, R. (1999). Teaching Strategies for Students with Brain Injuries. Wake Forest, NC: Lash and Associates Publishing/Training Inc.

Vaishnavi, S., Rao, V., and Fann, J. R. (2009). Neuropsychiatric Problems After Traumatic Brain Injury: Unraveling the Silent Epidemic. *Psychosomatics,* 50 (3), 198-205.

Van Reekum, R., Cohen, T., and Wong, J. (2000). Can traumatic brain injury cause psychiatric disorders? *The Journal of Neuropsychiatry and Clinical Neurosciences*, 12, 316-327.

Vygotsky, L. S. (1978). Mind in society: The development of higher psychological processes. Cambridge, MA: Harvard University Press.

Voytek, B. and Knight, R. T. (2010). Prefrontal cortex and basal ganglia contributions to visual working memory. *Proceedings of the National Academy of Sciences of the United States of America*, 107, 18167–18172.

Writer, B. W. and Schillerstrom, J. E. (2009). Psychopharmacological Treatment for Cognitive Impairment in Survivors of Traumatic Brain Injury: A Critical Review. *The Journal of Neuropsychiatry and Clinical Neurosciences,* 21, 362-370.

Zhang, L., Plotkin, R. C., Wang, G., Sandel, M. E., and Lee, S. (2004). Cholinergic augmentation with donepezil enhances recovery in short term memory and sustained attention after traumatic brain injury. *Archives of Physical Medicine and Rehabilitation*, 85, 1050–1055.

In: Research Trends in Behavior ...
Editor: Miao-Kun Sun

ISBN: 978-1-63485-461-0

Chapter 7

CEREBELLAR CONTRIBUTIONS TO IMPLICIT LEARNING AND EXECUTIVE FUNCTIONS

Brad Tyson, Psy.D., Crystal Lantrip, Ph.D. and Robert M. Roth, Ph.D.*
Neuropsychology Program and Brain Imaging Laboratory, Department of Psychiatry, Geisel School of Medicine at Dartmouth, Lebanon, NH, US

ABSTRACT

The cerebellum is increasingly recognized as a structure that regulates cognitive and emotional functioning in much the same way that it modulates motor activity. Reciprocal connections with prefrontal and temporoparietal association cortices facilitate cerebellar modulation of implicit learning and executive functions, while connections with paralimbic regions allow for cerebellar regulation of emotional responses. Furthermore, recent evidence indicates that the cerebellum is reciprocally connected with the basal ganglia, forming an interconnected subcortical network with an extensive influence on cortical processing. In this review, we first discuss the neuroanatomical basis of the cerebellum's role in implicit learning and executive functioning. Next, we examine

* Correspondence and requests for reprints: Robert M. Roth, Ph.D., Department of Psychiatry, Geisel School of Medicine at Dartmouth, One Medical Center Drive, Lebanon, NH 03756-0001. E-Mail: Robert.M.Roth@Dartmouth.edu

evidence of cerebellar contributions to executive dysfunction in select neurological and psychiatric illnesses. We conclude with a brief discussion regarding potential treatments targeting the cerebellum.

Keywords: cerebellum, executive function, emotion, implicit learning

1. Introduction

The essential function of the cerebellum was long considered to be the coordination of voluntary movement. Early observations of patients with cerebellar lesions described fragmentation of normal motor sequences (dysynergia) and of rapid alternating movements (dysdiadochokinesia), as well as deficits in the rate, range, and force of movement resulting in the overshooting or undershooting of intended targets (dysmetria) (Babinski, 1899; Holmes, 1939; Ropper and Samuels, 2009). The classical view of cerebrocerebellar connections is that the cerebellum receives input from select regions of the neocortex and projects this information back through the ventrolateral nucleus of the thalamus to the primary motor cortex. According to this view, cerebellar output influenced motor control and abnormal activity in this circuit would lead to purely motor deficits.

In the past several decades, the role of the cerebellum in the implicit learning and homeostatic regulation of both motor and non-motor information has been emphasized. Ito (2010) has argued that the cerebellum is involved in the adaptive control of activities that are performed outside of a person's conscious awareness, such as when a behavior becomes more refined due to practice. Importantly, this role was extended to cognitive processes. Specifically, he asserts that repetitious thoughts and mental plans become more implicit over time, that is, they require less and less conscious effort as the cerebellum forms an internal representation of the cortical mental model (Ito, 2010). Schmahmann (2000) proposed a *universal cerebellar transform* to describe the structure's all-encompassing role in establishing and maintaining behavior at an optimum level, effectively smoothing out performance in all domains. Furthermore, he has argued that the concept of *dysmetria of thought* is analogous with dysmetria of the motor system, providing a coherent model for explaining the impairments of higher-order behavior that result when the "distributed neural circuits subserving cognitive operations are deprived of cerebellar modulation" (Schmahmann, 1998; pp. 362). That is, the cerebellum regulates the speed, capacity, consistency and appropriateness of cognitive and emotional processes in much the same way as it regulates the rate, force, and accuracy of movements. The corresponding neuropsychological impairments of cerebellar dysfunction are related to exaggeration (overshoot) and diminution (undershoot) of responses to the internal or external environment, particularly in the domains of attention control, emotional regulation and social skill set (Schmahmann, Weilburg, and Sherman, 2007).

More recently, the idea of *embodied cognition* has reemerged, leading some researchers to suggest that the cognitive system evolved primarily to accommodate the motor system (Koziol, Budding, and Chidekel, 2012). Indeed, movement disorders associated with subcortical dysfunction often have a qualitatively similar cognitive correlate (see Table 1). For example, bradykinesia and rigidity, cardinal motor symptoms of Parkinson's disease (PD), are often accompanied by the cognitive features of reduced processing speed and perseveration. Choreathetosis, the primary hyperkinetic movement abnormality of Huntington's disease, is often accompanied by cognitive features such as impulsivity and distractibility. Contemporary analyses of cerebellar connectivity have also advanced our understanding of cerebellar functional neuroanatomy. It is now clear that efferents from the cerebellar nuclei project to multiple subnuclei of the thalamus, which then project to a myriad of association cortices. Moreover, recent findings have shown that the cerebellum and basal ganglia are densely interconnected (Bostan, Dum, and Strick, 2013). These neuroanatomical and clinical findings suggest that the cerebellum directly influences a wide range of both motor and non-motor activity.

Table 1. Cognitive mirroring of subcortical motor symptoms

Ranking of common movement disorders by speed[1]	Ranking of common cognitive symptoms by speed
Bradykinesia, hypokinesia	Bradyphrenia, decreased processing speed
Rigidity, dystonia	Perseveration, obsessional thinking
Athetosis, chorea, ballismus	Response inhibition, impulsivity
Tics, myoclonus	Distractibility

[1]Adapted from Blumenfeld, 2011.

In the present review, we first provide an overview of the functional neuroanatomy of the cerebellum. Next, we discuss contributions of the cerebellum to implicit learning and executive functioning in healthy individuals. We then provide examples of cerebellar contributions to executive dysfunction in select clinical populations. Finally, we briefly discuss recent research on potential treatments targeting the cerebellum and recommended directions for future research.

2. Functional Neuroanatomy of the Cerebellum

The neuroanatomy of the cerebellum and its connections with the rest of the brain provides a basis for understanding its role in executive functioning (for a more detailed review, see Blumenfeld, 2011; Haines, 2014). The surface anatomy of the cerebellum is comprised of a midline vermis that separates the structure into right and left cerebellar hemispheres. The anterior lobes, which comprise the most superior surface of the cerebellum, and the posterior lobes, which include much of the superior surface and the entire inferior surface, are separated horizontally by the primary fissure. The posterior lobe is the largest subdivision of the cerebellum in humans and is often referred to as the neocerebellum as its evolutionary expansion closely mirrored that of the prefrontal cortex. A deep horizontal fissure traverses the posterior lobe just below the primary fissure. The flocculonodular lobe, which is comprised of two flocculi connected by thin pedicles to the midline nodulus, is located on the ventral surface and separated horizontally from the posterior lobe by the posterolateral fissure. The cerebellar tonsils are clinically relevant as increased intracranial pressure may provoke downward herniation through the foramen magnum and cause death due to compression of medullary cardiorespiratory centers. Embryologically, the cerebellum is derived from the metencephalon and connected to the pons and the rest of the brain by the superior, middle and inferior cerebellar peduncles (Figure 1).

The cerebellum forms the roof of the fourth ventricle and is covered by small-ridged folia, rather than large gyri. A midsagittal section displays the beautiful branching white and grey matter pattern of the arbor vitae (see Figure 2).

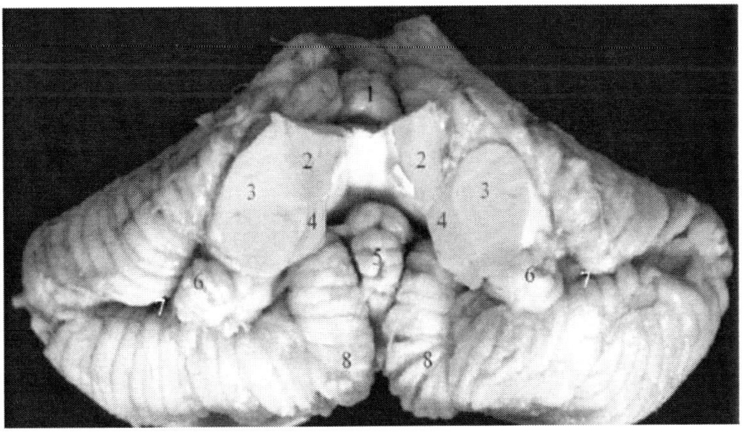

Figure 1. Ventral view with brainstem removed. Note: 1. Vermis. 2. Superior cerebellar peduncle (red). 3. Middle cerebellar peduncle (blue). 4. Inferior cerebellar peduncle (green). 5. Nodulus. 6. Flocculus. 7. Posterolateral fissure. 8. Cerebellar tonsils.

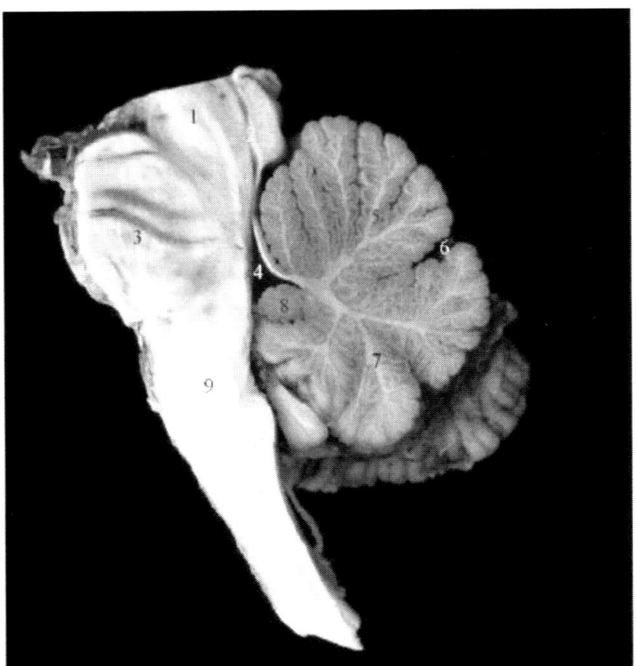

Figure 2. Midsagittal section showing the arbor vitae. Note: 1. Midbrain. 2. Cerebral aqueduct. 3. Pons. 4. Fourth ventricle. 5. Anterior lobe (red). 6. Primary fissure. 7. Posterior lobe (blue). 8. Nodulus (green). 9. Medulla.

A horizontal section showcases four deep cerebellar nuclei, represented bilaterally on each side of the midline, which relay all cerebellar output (see Figure 3). Lateral to medial, the deep cerebellar nuclei include the dentate, emboliform, globose, and fastigial nuclei. The dentate receives input from the lateral cerebellar hemispheres and projects to a variety of motor and non-motor cortical regions. The emboliform and globose nuclei are sometimes termed the interpositus nuclei as they are located between the dentate and fastigial nuclei and receive input from the intermediate cerebellar hemispheres. The fasigial nuclei receive information primarily from the vermis and project many efferents to limbic structures. The three-layered cerebellar cortex is uniformly composed of the molecular layer, the Purkinje cell layer and the granule cell layer. Because of the homogeneity of the cerebellar cortical circuitry, it has been suggested that the cerebellum performs the same general computations on all afferent information it receives (Ito, 1993).

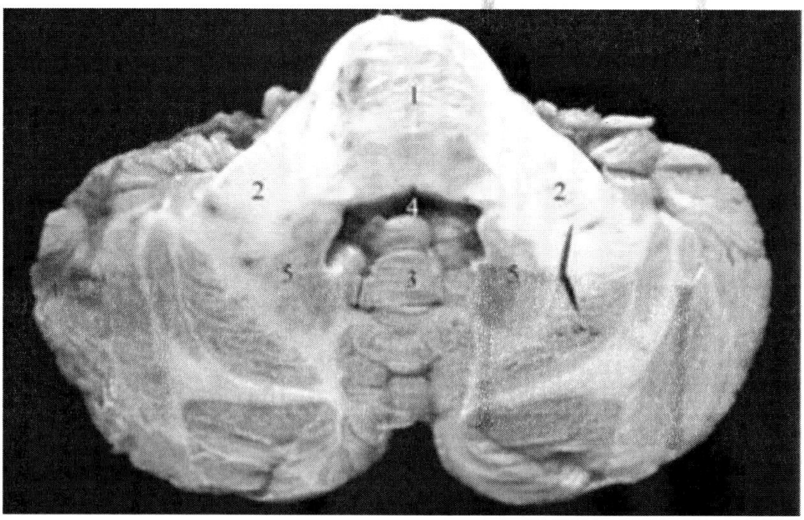

Figure 3. Cross section at level of caudal pons. Note: 1. Pons 2. Middle cerebellar peduncle. 3. Nodulus. 4. Fourth ventricle. 5. Deep cerebellar nuclei.

Cerebellar function can be organized anatomically along an anterior-posterior gradient and a medial-lateral gradient (Schmahmann and Pandya, 1997). These functional divisions provide valuable insight into the cognitive and emotional features of the cerebellum. The anterior-posterior gradient is composed of the anterior and posterior lobes (see Figure 4). The smaller flocculonodular lobe is located ventrally and important for equilibrium, balance and extraocular movements. The anterior lobe maintains body posture by modifying muscle tone and regulating voluntary movements. The anterior medial areas of the posterior lobe facilitate smooth, coordinated voluntary and skilled movements and ensure that the force, direction and distance are accurate. It also plays a critical role in motor learning and procedural memory. Inferior lateral areas of the posterior lobe are involved in diverse cognitive functions including attention, executive functioning, speech and language ability, and visuospatial skills. Thus, the anterior-posterior gradient suggests that lesions in the anterior lobes will generate sensorimotor deficits, while lesions of the posterior lobes will result in cognitive changes.

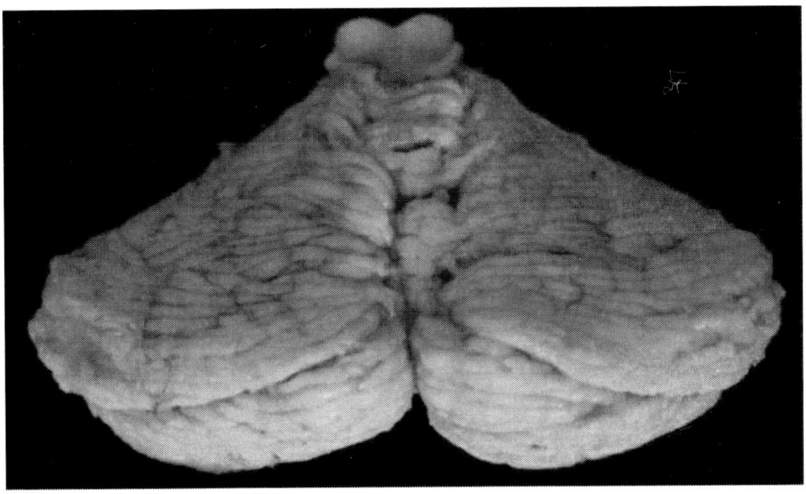

Figure 4. Anterior-posterior gradient. Note: The anterior lobe (red) is separated from the posterior lobe (blue) by the primary fissure. The deep horizontal fissure can be seen traversing the posterior lobe.

The medial-lateral gradient is composed of the vermian zone, the immediately adjacent intermediate or paravermian zone, and the lateral or hemispheric zone (see Figure 5). The anterior vermis and part of the posterior vermis are collectively referred to as the spinocerebellum, and exert a regulatory influence on posture and muscle tone. More posterior regions of the vermis have connections with reticular nuclei as well as the hippocampus, amygdala, hypothalamus, and cingulate gyrus and help regulate aspects of attention, emotion and autonomic functioning. Consequently, this region of the vermis is sometimes referred to as the limbic cerebellum. The intermediate zones bordering the vermis help coordinate proximal and trunk muscles controlling posture and gait. The lateral zones constitute the majority of the cerebellar hemispheres and are involved in planning, programming and coordination of the extremities. Posterior and inferior regions of the lateral zone are primarily involved in cognitive functions. Thus, the medial-lateral gradient suggests that lesions of medial cerebellar regions (vermian and intermediate zones) will generate sensorimotor deficits, while lesions to lateral regions will result in cognitive changes. If lesions involve posterior and inferior regions of the vermis, problems with emotional regulation may emerge.

It is also important to recognize the dense interconnectivity between the cerebellum and the rest of the brain. Cerebellar connections with the lateral motor system cross twice, once as outputs exit the deep cerebellar nuclei in the decussation of the superior cerebellar peduncle, and again as the corticospinal and rubrospinal tracts descend to the spinal cord. Thus, lesions of the cerebellar hemispheres cause ipsilateral motor deficits. Cerebrocerebellar connections only cross once in the decussation of the superior cerebellar peduncle, so lesions of the cerebellar hemispheres result in cognitive deficits typically associated with the contralateral hemisphere. For example, right cerebellar lesions may lead to impairments in aspects of language functioning, while left cerebellar lesions may lead to visuospatial problems.

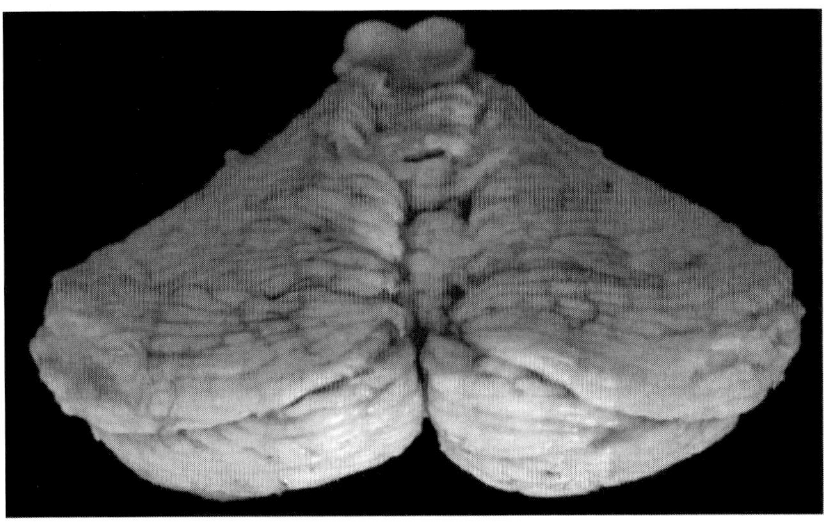

Figure 5. Medial-lateral gradient. Note: Vermian zone (red), paravermian or intermediate zone (green), lateral or hemispheric zone (blue).

The cerebellum regulates cortical information processing through cortico-ponto-cerebellar and cerebello-thalamo-cortical loops. Nearly all regions of the association cortex and paralimbic regions project to the pontine nuclei (Schmahmann and Pandya, 1997). The pontine nuclei send inputs through the middle cerebellar peduncle to the cerebellar cortex. This information is processed by internal cerebellar circuitry and projected to deep cerebellar nuclei, completing the cortico-ponto-cerebellar pathway or feed-forward limb. The deep cerebellar nuclei project through the superior cerebellar peduncle past the red nuclei to multiple subnuclei of thalamus, which relays information back to the cortical region where the circuit originated completing the cerebello-thalamo-cortical pathway or feedback limb. Thus, the cortico-ponto-cerebellar pathway provides cortical input to the cerebellum, which is modified and refined, and returned to the cerebral cortex through the cerebello-thalamo-cortical pathway.

Frontocerebellar circuits play an important role in a diversity of executive functions. Four topographically distinct frontocerebellar circuits have been identified. The first circuit projects to the motor cortex, the second to the dorsolateral prefrontal cortex, the third to the medial prefrontal cortex, and the fourth to the anterior prefrontal cortex (Krienen and Buckner, 2009). In humans the largest proportion of afferent fibers into the pontine nuclei and cerebellum originate from the dorsolateral prefrontal cortex (Ramnani et al., 2006). Therefore, cognitive impairments secondary to cerebellar disruption will most likely resemble those of the dorsolateral prefrontal cortex.

Another interconnected structure influencing cerebellar functioning is the inferior olivary nuclei of the medulla, which receives input from the red nucleus, zona incerta and deep cerebellar nuclei and projects olivocerebellar fibers to the contralateral cerebellar hemisphere through the inferior cerebellar peduncle. This olivocerebellar pathway appears to function as an error detection and correction system. It has been proposed that prefrontal influences on olivocerebellar circuits may help the cerebellum rapidly and efficiently switch between conscious control during skill acquisition and completely automatized behaviors involving previously mastered skills (Koziol et al., 2012).

Solidifying the changing views of cerebellar functional neuroanatomy are recent findings that the cerebellum and basal ganglia are reciprocally connected. Virus transport experiments have demonstrated that the dentate nucleus projects directly to the striatum, the primary input region of the basal ganglia, and that the subthalamic nucleus, a structure involved in behavioral inhibition, projects directly to the cerebellar cortex (Hoshi et al., 2005; Bostan, Dum, and Strick, 2010). These findings indicate that pathways from the dentate nucleus to the striatum enable an output from the cerebellum to influence the basal ganglia, and pathways from the subthalamic nucleus to the cerebellar cortex allows the output from the basal ganglia to influence functions within the cerebellum. Therefore, three main subcortical structures (thalamus, basal ganglia and cerebellum) appear to interact in such a way that abnormal activity in one structure has the potential to effect the subcortical system as a whole, which in turn, can have wide ranging effects on cortical functioning.

3. Neuropsychology of the Cerebellum

The cerebellum has been implicated in diverse neuropsychological functions such as attention, implicit learning, executive function, speech and language, visuospatial ability, as well as sensorimotor skills. Here, we provide an overview of cerebellar involvement in implicit learning and executive functioning. We then discuss evidence for a cerebellar contribution to executive dysfunction in a number of neurologic and psychiatric disorders.

4. Role of the Cerebellum in Implicit Learning

The cerebellum has been shown to be involved in the initial learning of sequences, detection and correction of errors in skill acquisition, coordination and timing of action sequences, anticipatory behavioral adjustments, and is theorized to regulate behavior through a more generalized error prediction and supervisory learning system (Bares et al., 2007; Doya, 2000; Dreher and Grafman, 2002; Koziol and Budding, 2009; Torriero et al., 2007). During skill acquisition, the cerebellum is theorized to create an internal representation of the cortical mental model, forming what has been referred to as a *forward model* of the brain's usual pattern of behavior, with neural traces hypothesized to be stored in prefrontal-posterior working memory networks (Higuchi, Imamizu, and Kawato, 2007; Ito, 2008).

Once this model is created, the cerebellum attempts to anticipate the outcome of an activity based on previous experiences. In other words, the cerebellum receives cortical input regarding current behavior and attempts to adapt this information to the imminent real-time context before sending back to the cortex. The cortex modifies behavior based on cerebellar feedback regarding the anticipated outcome. The olivocerebellar system detects errors in comparison to the model, codes the errors and helps further refine the model (Ito, 2013).

Through practice and repetition, a behavior becomes increasingly efficient and economic, eventually no longer requiring conscious control or input forming what is referred to as an *inverse model*. Everyday behavior is largely based on the automaticity of inverse models, though when context changes, behavior can be modified through the development of forward models and the interactions of forward and inverse models.

5. Role of the Cerebellum in Executive Functions

Executive function may be conceptualized as a collection of interrelated supervisory or higher level cognitive processes involved in the selection, execution, and monitoring of domain specific cognitive processes and motor responses, as well as emotional processing. Stated more generally, executive functions are concerned with the self-regulation of cognition, behavior, and emotion (Barkley, 2001; Gioia, Isquith, Guy, and Kenworthy, 2000; Stuss and Alexander, 2000). The efficient, automatic quality of implicit processes plays a significant role in the multidimensional construct of executive functions. These automatic behaviors are economic in familiar contexts and, by alternating with effortful higher order control, modifiable in anticipation of novel contextual changes. It has been suggested that the cerebellum modulates executive functioning by instructing the prefrontal cortex how to anticipate these contextual changes and potential outcomes (Koziol et al., 2012).

Studies of patients with neurodevelopmental or acquired abnormality of the cerebellum, as well as studies in such patients and healthy individuals employing a wide range of imaging techniques, such as structural and functional magnetic resonance imaging (MRI, fMRI) and positron emission tomography (PET), have implicated the cerebellum in a variety of executive functions. Here, we address working memory, verbal fluency, cognitive flexibility, inhibitory control, planning, problem solving and decision making, and emotion regulation.

5.1. Working Memory

A deficit in verbal working memory is one of the most consistently observed executive problems associated with cerebellar abnormality in humans, especially subsequent to disruption of the right cerebellar hemisphere (Bellebaum and Daum, 2007; Chen, Ho, and Desmond, 2014; Stoodley and Schmahmann, 2009). Drawing on Baddeley's (1992) classic model of working memory, Chen and Desmond hypothesized that the cerebellum has two anatomically distinct roles during verbal working memory: articulatory rehearsal, and phonological maintenance and storage (Chen and Desmond, 2005). Articulatory rehearsal has been reported to involve a loop between the right lateral cerebellar hemisphere and Broca's area, while maintenance and storage of phonological information involves a loop between the right posterolateral cerebellar hemisphere and the left inferior parietal lobule.

Marvel and Desmond (2010) similarly distinguish between motor and cognitive channels of cerebellar output in working memory. They also proposed that the cerebellum enhances verbal working memory by supporting inner speech mechanisms, which is consistent with studies showing involvement of medial regions of the anterior cerebellum in the control of motoric aspects of speech, and lateral portions of the anterior cerebellum in the support of speech planning and preparation (Durisko and Fiez, 2010). Indeed, the posterior inferior cerebellum is active when information is maintained across a delay, but this activation appears to be independent of speech itself and is likely related to phonological storage processes (Marvel and Desmond, 2010). Cerebellar influences on working memory provides the foundation for cerebellar contributions to executive functioning more generally and has a significant impact on related skills such as the initial learning of sequences, temporal ordering, mental rehearsal, context monitoring, and the anticipation of imminent events based upon previous experience.

5.2. Verbal Fluency

Performance on verbal fluency tasks has been linked to functioning of both posterolateral cerebellar hemispheres, though most consistently with the right posterolateral hemisphere, with greater involvement of the anterior lobe when articulation is required (Ackermann, Vogel, Petersen, and Poremba, 1992; Fiez and Raichle, 1997). Letter fluency tasks, involving the rapid generation of words to a letter cue (e.g., rapidly generating words beginning the letter F), may be more likely to involve the cerebellum than category fluency tasks (e.g., rapidly generating words in a given category such as animals), likely due to the stronger association of letter fluency tasks to prefrontal functioning (Schweizer, Alexander, Susan Gillingham, Cusimano, and Stuss, 2010). Structural MRI studies have shown a significant correlation between verbal fluency and grey matter density in the bilateral inferior cerebellum (Grogan, Green, Ali, Crinion, and Price, 2009). An fMRI study found that performance on verb generation tasks is associated with right posterolateral cerebellum activation (Frings et al., 2006). Of note, the left cerebellum has also been implicated in design fluency, though this has rarely been studied (Gottwald, Wilde, Mihajlovic, and Mehdorn, 2004). Research findings in this area suggest a strong lateralized cerebellar influence on verbal fluency, with anterior regions shaping motoric aspects of speech and posterior regions having a relative impact on the timing and generation of language.

5.3. Cognitive Flexibility

The cerebellum has been reported to contribute to cognitive flexibility, especially when novel problem solving or rapid set shifting is required. Early functional neuroimaging studies demonstrated activation in the left dorsolateral prefrontal cortex and right lateral cerebellum during performance of the Wisconsin Card Sort Test (Berman et al., 1995; Nagahama et al., 1996), with more recent work specifically implicating the posterior cerebellum in the set-shifting aspect of the task (Lie, Specht, Marshall, and Fink, 2006). An event-related potential study observed deficits in the ability to selectively shift attention in young participants with damage to the neocerebellum (Akshoomoff and Courchesne, 1994). Increased error rates in patients with cerebellar lesions have been reported on tasks requiring the shifting of attention between visual and auditory stimuli, as well as tasks involving simultaneous processing of visual and auditory stimuli (Gottwald et al., 2004; Ravizza and Ivry, 2001). Such increased error rates highlight the cerebellum's role in learning and performance efficiency during tasks involving aspects of cognitive flexibility.

Involvement of the cerebellum in cognitive flexibility appears consistent with the theory of internal models. That is, the ability to efficiently coordinate and shift attention between two or more tasks will likely be enhanced when one of the tasks can be performed automatically, allowing for more attention resources to be devoted to learning how to perform the other, non-automated task (Bellebaum and Daum, 2007). With practice and repetition, internal models are refined, leading to an improved ability to rapidly process multiple sources of information sequentially, selectively and simultaneously. Ineffective cerebellar modulation of the dorsolateral prefrontal cortex can lead to a decreased efficiency in these abilities. Thus, these findings suggest that the cerebellum influences cognitive flexibility through its role in the working memory and possibly by switching between forward and inverse models during task performance.

5.4. Inhibitory Control

Functional neuroimaging studies using tasks that require inhibition of a response have frequently observed activation of the cerebellum. For example, in one fMRI study, participants completed a random number generation task in which they were asked to silently generate random sequences of single digit numbers in synchrony with a pacing stimulus without repeating, numerically sequencing, or producing numbers according to special schemes such as counting by two's (Daniels, Witt, Wolff, Jansen, and Deuschl, 2003). During an initial set of trials involving random number generation every second, activation was observed bilaterally in the prefrontal and posterior parietal cortices, more prominently on left, as well as in the posterior cerebellar hemispheres, though more prominent on the right. During a more difficult second condition involving generation of two numbers every second, there was less activity in prefrontal and parietal cortices and no significant activity in the cerebellum. The authors concluded that the cognitive processes responsible for inhibitory control during the second condition were less active to maintain the increased rate of number generation. A recent fMRI study investigating the neural correlates of verbal and visuospatial versions of the Stroop test found small regions of activation common to both tasks, including the bilateral anterior cingulate cortices, left frontal parietal cortex and right cerebellum (Zoccatelli, Beltramello, Alessandrini, Pizzini, and Tassinari, 2010). These findings suggest that the cerebellum influences response inhibition through the structure's role in the regulation of timing functions, such as temporal ordering and event sequencing.

5.5. Planning

The cerebellum has long been recognized as a crucial part of a distributed frontal-subcortical network involved in motor planning, modulation and execution. This provides a useful heuristic for understanding the cerebellum's role in cognitive planning. In an important early study in this area, patients with pure cerebellar atrophy (no extracerebellar damage) demonstrated significant difficulty on the Tower of Hanoi, a classic neuropsychological test of planning (Grafman et al., 1992). Patients solved significantly less problems overall, had longer mean first move times (a measure of planning efficiency) and made more rule violations than controls. There was no significant relationship between age, education, global motor or cognitive impairment, depression, learning or verbal fluency and the number of problems solved on the Tower of Hanoi. Functional neuroimaging has demonstrated activation of the left cerebellum during performance on the Tower of London task, likely reflecting the prominent visuospatial demands of such tasks (Beauchamp, Dagher, Aston, and Doyon, 2003; Schall et al., 2003). The left cerebellum has also been implicated in other tasks involving visuospatial planning and problem solving such as chess, as well as the strategy taken to copy a complex abstract geometric figure (Atherton, Zhuang, Bart, Hu, and He, 2003; Gottwald et al., 2004). Overall, these and related findings suggest that the cerebellum influences aspects of planning through the anticipation and prediction of motor and non-motor outcomes.

5.6. Problem Solving and Decision Making

A growing body of research has implicated the cerebellum in problem solving and decision making. An fMRI study that employed a probabilistic reasoning task provided evidence that the neocerebellum helps mediate the probabilistic inferences that guide decision making under conditions of uncertainty (Blackwood et al., 2004). The authors hypothesized that the neocerebellum constructs internal representations of uncertain events, and that such probabilistic models improve the cerebellum's predictive capacity in novel contexts.

Another study employed PET during a computerized gambling card game assessing the ability to weigh short-term rewards against long-term losses (Ernst et al., 2002). Decision making was found to be associated with activation of the orbital and dorsolateral prefrontal cortices, anterior cingulate gyrus, insula, inferior parietal cortex, thalamus (predominantly on the right side), and lateral regions of the cerebellum (predominantly on the left side). Recruitment of the cerebellum was related to both decision making and the use of a learned strategy. The authors interpreted their findings as suggesting that the cerebellum plays an important role in error-based learning and the processing of error signals necessary for assessing risk and improving decision making.

A recent fMRI study of problem solving compared "aha" experiences defined as successful responses to novel and interesting riddles, with "no aha" experiences defined as responses to boring and easily solved riddles (Qiu et al., 2010). Results implicated a problem solving network that included the left inferior and middle frontal cortex, precuneus, inferior occipital lobe and bilateral areas of the posterior cerebellum. The authors concluded that the cerebellum contributes to the rapid deployment of attentional resources that serve to amplify information necessary for novel problem solving. Overall, these and related findings suggest that the cerebellum influences aspects of problem solving and decision making through its role in the initial learning of novel information, anticipation and prediction, and working memory.

5.7. Emotion Regulation

A recent meta-analysis of neuroimaging studies found that prefrontal-parietal-cerebellar circuits are more active during emotion and cognitive tasks than action execution tasks (Balsters, Laird, Fox, and Eickhoff, 2013). Indeed, the cerebellum has been implicated in the processing and regulation of emotion during tasks such as viewing emotional images, facial expressions and humorous images, identifying prosody, simulating mood states, anticipating pain and empathy towards another's pain, fear conditioning and the processing of threatening cues (Bartolo et al., 2006; Fusar-Poli et al., 2009; Singer et al., 2004; Stoodley and Schmahmann, 2009; Turner et al., 2007). A recent study found cerebellar vermis and hemisphere activation during the viewing of images rated as disgusting and posterior cerebellar activation to pictures evoking happiness; cerebellar connectivity with limbic regions was observed during the viewing of both picture types (Schienle and Scharmuller, 2013). Functional neuroimaging studies have also observed cerebellar activation when participants were required to decrease their emotional response to pleasant and unpleasant visual stimuli (Seo et al., 2013). These findings suggest that the cerebellum likely contributes to emotional regulation through homeostatic regulation and timing of appropriate responses.

6. The Cerebellum in Neurological and Psychiatric Disorders

Cerebellar contributions to implicit learning and executive function deficits have been increasingly implicated in a variety of neurological and psychiatric disorders. In particular, the role of the cerebellum in working memory and verbal fluency has broad clinical implications including disruptions in language acquisition during childhood, unchecked inner speech involved in psychiatric disorders, and attentional impairments following acquired cerebellar lesions. Localized dysfunction may lead to limited motor or non-motor deficits, particular if these lesions are acquired later in life. More widespread cerebellar dysfunction has extensive effects on implicit learning and executive functioning and this is particularly true in the case of neurodevelopmental and congenital cerebellar abnormalities. Because the sequelae of acquired cerebellar disruption in adulthood are often subtle, the cognitive and emotional effects may be more difficult to identify than the more obvious motor disturbances. In this section, we provide examples of cerebellar involvement and executive dysfunction in select neurological and psychiatric disorders.

7. Cerebellar Tumors

Resection of tumors in the cerebellar hemispheres or vermis, as well as paraneoplastic cerebellar degeneration, have been reported to be associated with executive dysfunction (Aarsen, Van Dongen, Paquier, Van Mourik, and Catsman-Berrevoets, 2004; Collinson, Anthonisz, Courtenay, and Winter, 2006; Karatekin, Lazareff, and Asarnow, 2000; Levisohn, Cronin-Golomb, and Schmahmann, 2000; Vaquero, Gomez, Quintero, Gonzalez-Rosa, and Marquez, 2008). The *posterior fossa syndrome* is sometimes observed in children following resection of posterior fossa tumors and involves a constellation of neuropsychological symptoms including transient mutism, executive dysfunction, and behavioral abnormalities. Affective changes are also observed in relation to this syndrome, such as apathy, withdrawal, irritability, excessive laughing and agitation (De Smet et al., 2009). In some children with posterior fossa tumors, however, executive dysfunction has been reported to be associated with cranial radiation therapy (Copeland, deMoor, Moore, and Ater, 1999). The *cerebellar cognitive affective syndrome* is a constellation of affective, executive, linguistic, and visuospatial changes occurring most commonly in patients with lesions of the posterior lobe of the cerebellum and vermis (Schmahmann and Sherman, 1998). Impairments in executive function have included difficulties with planning, set-shifting, abstract reasoning, working memory and verbal fluency. Personality change has also been reported, including blunting of affect as well as disinhibited and inappropriate behavior. Such changes are consistent with recent work that has observed generally normal emotion identification, but impaired cognitive control over emotions, in children with cerebellar tumors (Hopyan, Laughlin, and Dennis, 2010).

8. Autism Spectrum Disorders

A possible role for the cerebellum in autism spectrum disorders (ASD) has been the subject of intensive research in recent years (Fatemi et al., 2012). Structural abnormality of the region has been observed in post-mortem tissue samples (Schmitz and Rezaie, 2008) and on structural MRI scans of grey and white matter (Ecker et al., 2012; Scott, Schumann, Goodlin-Jones, and Amaral, 2009; Sivaswamy et al., 2010), including diffusion tensor imaging evidence suggesting reduced Purkinje cell fibers (Jeong, Tiwari, Behen, Chugani, and Chugani, 2014). In addition, ample evidence has accumulated for the presence of executive dysfunction in ASD through performance-based measures and parent rating of executive functions in everyday life (Chan et al., 2009; Kenworthy, Yerys, Anthony, and Wallace, 2008; Beatriz Luna, Doll, Hegedus, Minshew, and Sweeney, 2007; Rosenthal et al., 2013). Functional MRI studies have observed abnormalities in those with ASD during performance of executive function tasks involving random response generation (Gilbert, Bird, Brindley, Frith, and Burgess, 2008) and spatial working memory (Luna et al., 2002).

9. Attention Deficit Hyperactivity Disorder

Several authors have posited a role for the cerebellum in the etiology of attention-deficit/hyperactivity disorder (ADHD), including its involvement in executive and other cognitive deficits associated with the disorder (Krain and Castellanos, 2006; Roth and Saykin, 2004; Seidman, Valera, and Makris, 2005). Structural MRI studies have observed reduced cerebellar volume in the disorder (Berquin et al., 1998; Bledsoe, Semrud-Clikeman, and Pliszka, 2011; Castellanos et al., 2002; Makris et al., 2013; Mostofsky, Reiss, Lockhart, and Denckla, 1998), as well as an association between reduced volume and poorer performance on a cognitive flexibility task (McAlonan et al., 2009). Functional neuroimaging studies have shown abnormal cerebellar activation in ADHD during a variety of executive function tasks including those tapping working memory (Massat et al., 2012; Valera, Faraone, Biederman, Poldrack, and Seidman, 2005; Wolf et al., 2009), sustained attention and executive control (Wang et al., 2013), fluid reasoning (Tamm and Juranek, 2012), as well as time discrimination (Vloet et al., 2010).

Interestingly, atypical fMRI activation of frontocerebellar circuitry was observed during a forethought task in unaffected parents of children with ADHD (Rapin, Poissant, and Mendrek, 2014). This latter finding provides further evidence that cerebellar abnormality in the disorder is not due to secondary factors (e.g., medication exposure).

10. Tourette's Syndrome

Long considered a disorder of cortico-striato-thalamo-cortical circuits, recent research has implicated the cerebellum in motor and vocal tic generation in Tourette's syndrome (TS). Using PET, Lerner, et al., (2007) differentiated individuals with TS from controls by an abnormal metabolic pattern involving increased cerebellar and decreased basal ganglia metabolism. This study showed prominent activation of the cerebellum and insula during tic release. Tobe, et al. (2010) demonstrated reduced cerebellar hemisphere volume bilaterally on MRI in TS relative to controls. The degree of volume reduction in the most anterolateral cerebellar lobules was associated with more severe tic symptoms. Interestingly, relative hypertrophy of this region was seen in patients who had comorbid obsessive compulsive disorder (OCD) compared to those having TS without OCD, and greater hypertrophy was associated with more severe OCD symptoms. The authors theorized that reduced local cerebellar volumes and disruption of corticocerebellar regulatory loops may increase excitability of motor circuits and thereby worsen motor tics. They also proposed that superior portions of the cerebellar hemispheres are inhibitory regulators of language control and thus persons with TS may be impaired in their capacity to encode phonetic information though impaired phonetic storage (with contributions from anterolateral cerebellar hemispheres) and impaired subvocal rehearsal (with contributions from posterolateral cerebellar hemispheres), which could in turn disrupt language processing and impair the inhibition of spontaneous language generation.

11. Obsessive-Compulsive Disorder

The cerebellum has not received major attention in studies of OCD. As with TS, OCD is largely considered a disorder cortico-striato-thalamo-cortical circuitry, in particular, orbitofronto-striatal loops (Menzies, et al., 2008), and there is evidence of both executive dysfunction (for a review, see Roth, Lavoie, Mason, and O'Connor, 2013) and abnormal implicit learning /procedural memory (Kathmann, Rupertseder, Hauke, and Zaudig, 2005; Roth, Baribeau, Milovan, O'Connor, and Todorov, 2004) in the disorder. Roth et al. (2007) investigated the neural substrates of response inhibition in adults with OCD using a go/no-go task during fMRI. Positive correlations between brain activation and total symptom severity were found for the precuneus bilaterally, the right inferior temporal, postcentral and lingual gyri, the left inferior parietal lobule and left thalamus, as well as the right cerebellum. Anticevic et al. (2014) examined resting-state functional connectivity data in 27 patients with OCD and 66 healthy controls. Analysis revealed clusters of decreased connectivity in the left lateral prefrontal cortex. Increased global brain connectivity was seen in the dorsal striatum, anterior thalamus, right putamen and left cerebellar cortex. Cerebellar and striatal hyperconnectivity was modulated by medication status. Relative to unmedicated patients, those treated with selective serotonin reuptake inhibitors (SSRI's) showed better connectivity in the striatum and cerebellum indicating that pharmacotherapy may help modulate this circuitry.

12. Major Depressive Disorder

Neuropsychological studies have often observed impairments on tests of executive functions in major depressive disorder (MDD) (Snyder, 2013). Structural neuroimaging studies have observed cerebellar abnormality in MDD, albeit inconsistently (Peng et al., 2011; Pillay et al., 1997; Shah et al., 1992; Yucel et al., 2013). In contrast, the cerebellum has been commonly reported to be abnormal in functional neuroimaging studies of depression (Fitzgerald, Laird, Maller, and Daskalakis, 2008). These have mainly examined responses to emotional stimuli, such as emotional faces, with findings indicating abnormal activation to displays of a variety of emotions in patients with MDD. Furthermore, individuals at risk for developing MDD by virtue of having a high level of neuroticism also show abnormal cerebellar response to emotional stimuli (Chan, Norbury, Goodwin, and Harmer, 2009). Few studies, however, have directly reported on the association between cerebellar activation and performance on executive function tasks. In one such study, however, abnormally increased frontocerebellar connectivity was observed during performance of an fMRI working memory task (Vasic, Walter, Sambataro, and Wolf, 2009).

Consistent with findings in patients with MDD, other lines of evidence support a role for the cerebellum in emotional dysregulation. In particular, pathological laughter and crying has been linked to an abnormal cerebellum in patients with multiple system atrophy (Parvizi, Joseph, Press, and Schmahmann, 2007), and attributed to disruption of cerebro-ponto-cerebellar pathways resulting in a failure of cerebellar structures to automatically adjust the execution of laughter or crying to the context (Parvizi, Anderson, Martin, Damasio, and Damasio, 2001).

13. Schizophrenia

Several studies have implicated the cerebellum in the etiology of psychiatric symptoms and cognitive dysfunction associated with schizophrenia (Andreasen, Nopoulos, O'Leary, Miller, Wassink, and Flaum, 1999; Andreasen and Pierson, 2008; Picard, Amado, Mouchet-Mages, Olie, and Krebs, 2008). These have been supported by structural neuroimaging studies that have observed changes in both gray matter (Kuhn, Romanowski,

Schubert, and Gallinat, 2012; Rasser et al., 2010; Segarra et al., 2008) and white matter (Filippi et al., 2014; Koch et al., 2010) integrity in the disorder, as well as in first episode psychosis (Watson et al., 2012), indicating that medications cannot account for the findings. Structural abnormalities of the cerebellum have also been found to correlate with performance on tests of executive functions in patients with schizophrenia. For example, Segarra et al. (2008) reported that working memory dysfunctions in schizophrenia was associated with reduced grey matter in both cerebellar hemispheres and vermis, while cognitive flexibility was related to reduced cerebellar white matter volume bilaterally. Kuhn and colleagues (2012) reported that reduced grey matter volume in the left cerebellum was correlated with performance on part B of the Trail Making Test, which requires rapid visuomotor processing and cognitive flexibility, as well as with thought disorder. The authors interpreted their findings as supporting a role for the cerebellum in failure to adequately coordinate mental processes in schizophrenia.

Functional imaging studies of the resting-state have reported abnormal patterns of functional connectivity involving several regions of the cerebellum including the midbrain, thalamus and frontal cortex (Chen et al., 2013; Khadka et al., 2013). Abnormal connectivity of the dorsolateral prefrontal cortex with several regions including the cerebellum was observed in patients and in unaffected first-degree relatives of those with schizophrenia (Su et al., 2013). This abnormal connectivity was associated with performance on tasks of executive functions. Furthermore, in a recent review of fMRI studies of schizophrenia by Longu et al. (2012), almost two-thirds of studies found cerebellar hypoactivation during task performance (though this was associated in part to the age of participants), especially in the medial portion of the anterior lobe and the lateral hemispheres. In particular, a growing body of fMRI studies have observed abnormal activation of the cerebellum during executive function tasks, especially those involving working memory (Meyer-Lindenberg et al., 2005; Schlosser et al., 2003; White, Schmidt, Kim, and Calhoun, 2011).

14. Cerebellar Stroke

Executive dysfunction and emotional changes have been reported secondary to strokes involving the vascular territory of the posterior inferior cerebellar artery (PICA) and to a lesser extent the superior cerebellar artery

(Exner, Weniger, and Irle, 2004; Kalashnikova, Zueva, Pugacheva, and Korsakova, 2005; Manes, Villamil, Ameriso, Roca, and Torralva, 2009; Marien et al., 2009; Richter et al., 2007; Turner, et al., 2007; Yang, Kim, Lee, and Kim, 2007). Greater involvement of PICA territory subserving the posterior and inferior portions of the vermis is also commonly associated with affective changes. Impairments may follow a lateralized pattern, with right sided lesions precipitating the most significant cognitive changes in abilities such as verbal fluency and verbal working memory (Exner et al., 2004; Hokkanen, Kauranen, Roine, Salonen, and Kotila, 2006; Richter, et al., 2007; Schmahmann and Sherman, 1998). Interestingly, patients with cerebellar stroke have been observed to show greater activation outside of the cortico-cerebellar network during an fMRI working memory task, suggesting that stroke in the cerebellum has a significant impact on the functional integrity of other brain regions (Ziemus et al., 2007).

15. Parkinson's Disease

The cerebellum has often been overlooked in the study of PD, though there is a wealth of evidence implicating the structure in motor and non-motor features of the disease. Research has supported a unique role for the cerebellum in parkinsonian tremor, and deep brain stimulation (DBS) of the subthalamic nucleus may help normalize cerebellar functioning (Geday et al., 2009; Hilker et al., 2004; Bostan et al., 2013). Camicioli et al. (2009) assessed executive functions in PD with tests of working memory, inhibitory control, and cognitive flexibility and found significant correlations between executive functioning and grey matter atrophy in the middle temporal gyri, left precuneus, bilateral caudate and cerebellum. Using PET, Huang et al. (2007) found that memory and executive dysfunction in PD was associated with reduced metabolism in frontal and parietal association areas, and increases in the cerebellar vermis and dentate nuclei. Unlike the metabolic pattern in PD related motor impairment, this cognitive pattern was not significantly altered by treatment with either intravenous levodopa or DBS. The authors suggested that hypermetabolism in the cerebellum might reflect a compensatory effort to maintain cognitive function in PD.

16. Emerging Treatments Targeting the Cerebellum

As the cerebellum has been increasingly recognized as contributing to the cognitive and affective problems in a variety of disorders, researchers have begun to target the structure in investigations of treatment efforts. The motor features of cerebellar dysfunction have long been the target of therapeutic interventions by physical and occupational therapists. There is limited research regarding cognitive rehabilitation for the cognitive sequelae of cerebellar dysfunction, though improvements in sustained attention, planning, and organization have been reported using approaches based on cognitive behavioral therapy (Schweizer et al., 2008). Pharmacologic approaches to cerebellar behavioral alterations are currently based on a symptomatic approach, such as the treatment of mood, anxiety, or psychotic disorders. As noted above, there is evidence that SSRI's may help modulate cerebellar circuitry in OCD. However, more research is needed in this area. DBS may be helpful in normalizing aspects of cerebellar functioning through effects of thalamic and basal ganglia targets. Newer advances in neural stimulation also hold promise for treatment of cerebellar dysfunction.

Repetitive transcranial magnetic stimulation (rTMS) of the cerebellum has been shown to modulate the connectivity between the structure and the primary motor cortex, altering cerebellar excitability, but also as having more remote effects. For example, a PET study observed that rTMS of the left lateral cerebellum modulated the excitability of several brain regions involved in cognition and emotion including the prefrontal cortex (Cho et al., 2012). Such findings have led to the use of the procedure to assess the integrity of cerebello-thalamo-cortical circuitry and to evaluate the role of the cerebellum in non-motor processes in healthy and clinical populations (Grimaldi et al., 2014; Koch, 2010).

A number of studies have examined the effects of cerebellar rTMS on mood and emotion processing. In the first such study, rTMS of the medial but not lateral cerebellum resulted in improved mood and alertness in a sample of healthy adults (Schutter, van Honk, d'Alfonso, Peper, and Panksepp, 2003). In a follow-up study by this same research group, healthy adults received rTMS of the medial cerebellar, occipital lobe, and sham stimulation on three separate days (Schutter and van Honk, 2009). The effects of rTMS were assessed using self-reported mood during an emotion regulation task in which participants either looked at aversive or neutral scenes, or suppressed negative feelings experienced during the scenes. Results indicated that only cerebellar rTMS induced a significant increase in negative mood following the emotion regulation task. In a third study of healthy participants, the authors found that rTMS over the medial cerebellum was associated with increases in emotional responses to masked happy facial expressions, but not neutral or fearful expressions, though no changes in subjective mood ratings were observed (Schutter, Enter, and Hoppen-brouwers, 2009). Finally, in patients with schizophrenia, rTMS applied to the vermis was reported to reduce anergia and thought disorder in a case study (Garg, Tikka, Goyal, Sinha, and Nizamie, 2013), and yielded improvement on measures of happiness, sadness, alertness and energy, as well as amelioration on tests of attention, working memory, and visuospatial skills in a small sample (Demirtas-Tatlidede et al., 2010).

To our knowledge, no study to date has directly evaluated the effect of rTMS to the cerebellum in MDD. Stimulation of the left dorsolateral prefrontal cortex has, however, been associated with improved mood and increased regional cerebral blood flow in the cerebellum in a sample of patients having a mood disorder (Speer et al., 2000). In addition, rTMS of the left dorsolateral prefrontal cortex was reported to improve mood and alter fMRI activation in the cerebellum during the processing of emotional stimuli in patients with PD (Cardoso et al., 2008). Together, these findings provide further evidence for the involvement of the cerebellum in mood regulation.

CONCLUSION

The cerebellum has historically been viewed as a structure concerned with the coordination and control of movement. Our understanding of cerebellar functional neuroanatomy continues to evolve and recent findings of direct pathways between the cerebellum and basal ganglia ensure that this will continue to be a productive area of future research. Initially controversial, the role of the cerebellum in cognitive and emotional functioning can no longer be denied. Just as the cerebellum informs motor regions about the most efficient way to execute a motor response, it also informs prefrontal, parietal and paralimbic cortices how to manipulate ideas for successful execution of cognitive and emotional responses. A variety of theoretical models have been proposed to explain the cerebellum's influence on motor and non-motor functioning, though no single model has been universally accepted. Several lines of research have demonstrated an important role for this structure in implicit learning and executive functions in healthy individuals, as well as being implicated in a range of developmental and acquired illnesses. Accordingly, future investigations will be needed to develop neuropsychological tests sensitive to cerebellar dysfunction, advanced imaging techniques assessing in vivo cerebellar function and connectivity, multidisciplinary treatment approaches targeting cerebellar disruption, and eventually therapeutic interventions aimed at the prevention of cerebellar disease.

ACKNOWLEDGMENTS

Thank you to William Hickey, M.D. and Ekrem Maloku, M.D., Department of Pathology, Dartmouth-Hitchcock Medical Center, for providing the cerebellum images for this chapter.

REFERENCES

Aarsen, F. K., Van Dongen, H. R., Paquier, P. F., Van Mourik, M., and Catsman-Berrevoets, C. E. (2004). Long-term sequelae in children after cerebellar astrocytoma surgery. *Neurology,* 62(8), 1311-1316.

Ackermann, H., Vogel, M., Petersen, D., and Poremba, M. (1992). Speech deficits in ischaemic cerebellar lesions. *Journal of Neurology*, 239(4), 223-227.

Akshoomoff, N. A., and Courchesne, E. (1994). ERP evidence for a shifting attention deficit in patients with damage to the cerebellum. *Journal of Cognitive Neuroscience,* 6(4), 388-399.

Andreasen, N. C., Nopoulos, P., O'Leary, D. S., Millcr, D. D., Wassink, T., and Flaum, M. (1999). Defining the phenotype of schizophrenia: cognitive dysmetria and its neural mechanisms. *Biological Psychiatry*, 46(7), 908-920.

Andreasen, N. C., and Pierson, R. (2008). The role of the cerebellum in schizophrenia. *Biological Psychiatry*, 64(2), 81-88.

Anticevic, A., Hu, S., Zhang, S., Savic, A., Billingslea, E., Wasylink, S., Repovs, G., Cole, M.W., Bednarski, S., Krystal, J.H., Bloch, M.H., Li, C.S., and Pittenger, C. (2014). Global resting-state functional magnetic resonance imaging analysis identifies frontal cortex, striatal, and cerebellar dysconnectivity in obsessive-compulsive disorder. *Biological Psychiatry,* 75(8), 595-605.

Atherton, M., Zhuang, J., Bart, W. M., Hu, X., and He, S. (2003). A functional MRI study of high-level cognition. I. The game of chess. *Brain Research: Cognitive Brain Research,*16(1), 26-31.

Babinski, J. (1899). De l'asynergie cérébelleuse. *Revue Neurologique*, 7, 806-816.

Baddeley, A. (1992). Working memory. *Science*, 255(5044), 556-559.

Balsters, J. H., Laird, A. R., Fox, P. T., and Eickhoff, S. B. (2013). Bridging the gap between functional and anatomical features of cortico-cerebellar circuits using meta-analytic connectivity modeling. *Human Brain* Mapping.

Bares, M., Lungu, O., Liu, T., Waechter, T., Gomez, C. M., and Ashe, J. (2007). Impaired predictive motor timing in patients with cerebellar disorders. *Experimental Brain Research*, 180(2), 355-365.

Barkley, R. A. (2001). The executive functions and self-regulation: An evolutionary neuropsychological perspective. *Neuropsychology Review,* 11(1), 1-29.

Bartolo, A., Benuzzi, F., Nocetti, L., Baraldi, P., and Nichelli, P. (2006). Humor comprehension and appreciation: An fMRI study. *Journal of Cognitive Neuroscience*, 18(11), 1789-1798.

Beauchamp, M. H., Dagher, A., Aston, J. A., and Doyon, J. (2003). Dynamic functional changes associated with cognitive skill learning of an adapted version of the Tower of London task. *Neuroimage*, 20(3), 1649-1660.

Bellebaum, C., and Daum, I. (2007). Cerebellar involvement in executive control. *Cerebellum*, 6(3), 184-192.

Berman, K. F., Ostrem, J. L., Randolph, C., Gold, J., Goldberg, T. E., Coppola, R., Carson, R.E., Herscovitch, P., and Weinberger, D. R. (1995). Physiological activation of a cortical network during performance of the Wisconsin Card Sorting Test: A positron emission tomography study. *Neuropsychologia*, 33(8), 1027-1046.

Berquin, P. C., Giedd, J. N., Jacobsen, L. K., Hamburger, S. D., Krain, A. L., Rapoport, J. L., and Castellanos, F. X. (1998). Cerebellum in attention-deficit hyperactivity disorder: A morphometric MRI study. *Neurology*, 50(4), 1087-1093.

Blackwood, N., Ffytche, D., Simmons, A., Bentall, R., Murray, R., and Howard, R. (2004). The cerebellum and decision making under uncertainty. *Cognitive Brain Research*, 20(1), 46-53.

Bledsoe, J. C., Semrud-Clikeman, M., and Pliszka, S. R. (2011). Neuroanatomical and neuropsychological correlates of the cerebellum in children with attention-deficit/hyperactivity disorder-combined type. *Journal of the American Academy of Child and Adolescent Psychiatry*, 50(6), 593-601.

Blumenfeld, H. (2011). *Neuroanatomy Through Clinical Cases* (2 ed.). Sunderland, MA: Sinauer Associates, Inc.

Bostan, A. C., Dum, R. P., and Strick, P. L. (2013). Cerebellar networks with the cerebral cortex and basal ganglia. *Trends in Cognitive Sciences*, 17(5), 241-254.

Bostan, A. C., Dum, R. P., and Strick, P. L. (2010). The basal ganglia communicate with the cerebellum. *Proceedings of the National Academy of Sciences*, 107(18), 8452-8456.

Camicioli, R., Gee, M., Bouchard, T. P., Fisher, N. J., Hanstock, C. C., Emery, D. J., and Martin, W. R. (2009). Voxel-based morphometry reveals extra-nigral atrophy patterns associated with dopamine refractory cognitive and motor impairment in parkinsonism. *Parkinsonism and Related Disorders*, 15(3), 187-195.

Cardoso, E. F., Fregni, F., Martins Maia, F., Boggio, P. S., Luis Myczkowski, M., Coracini, K., Lopes Vieira, A., Melo, L.M., Sato, J.R., Antonio Marcolin, M., Rigonatti, S.P., Cruz, A.C. Jr, Reis Barbosa, E., and Amaro, E., Jr. (2008). rTMS treatment for depression in Parkinson's disease increases BOLD responses in the left prefrontal cortex. *International Journal of Neuropsychopharmacology*, 11(2), 173-183.

Castellanos, F. X., Lee, P. P., Sharp, W., Jeffries, N. O., Greenstein, D. K., Clasen, L. S., Blumenthal, J.D., James, R.S., Ebens, C.L., Walter, J.M., Zijdenbos, A., Evans, A.C., Giedd, J.N., and Rapoport, J. L. (2002). Developmental trajectories of brain volume abnormalities in children and adolescents with attention-deficit/hyperactivity disorder. *Journal of the American Medical Association,* 288(14), 1740-1748.

Chan, A. S., Cheung, M. C., Han, Y. M., Sze, S. L., Leung, W. W., Man, H. S., and To, C. Y. (2009). Executive function deficits and neural discordance in children with autism spectrum disorders. *Clinical Neurophysiology*, 120(6), 1107-1115.

Chan, S. W., Norbury, R., Goodwin, G. M., and Harmer, C. J. (2009). Risk for depression and neural responses to fearful facial expressions of emotion. *British Journal of Psychiatry*, 194(2), 139-145.

Chen, S. H., and Desmond, J. E. (2005). Cerebrocerebellar networks during articulatory rehearsal and verbal working memory tasks. *Neuroimage,* 24(2), 332-338.

Chen, Y. L., Tu, P. C., Lee, Y. C., Chen, Y. S., Li, C. T., and Su, T. P. (2013). Resting-state fMRI mapping of cerebellar functional dysconnections involving multiple large-scale networks in patients with schizophrenia. *Schizophrenia Research,* 149(1-3), 26-34.

Chen, S. H., Ho, M.H., and Desmond, J. E. (2014). A meta-analysis of cerebellar contributions to higher cognition from PET and fMRI studies. *Human Brain Mapping*, 35 (2), 593-615.

Cho, S. S., Yoon, E. J., Bang, S. A., Park, H. S., Kim, Y. K., Strafella, A. P., and Kim, S. E. (2012). Metabolic changes of cerebrum by repetitive transcranial magnetic stimulation over lateral cerebellum: a study with FDG PET. *Cerebellum*, 11(3), 739-748.

Collinson, S. L., Anthonisz, B., Courtenay, D., and Winter, C. (2006). Frontal executive impairment associated with paraneoplastic cerebellar degeneration: A case study. *Neurocase,* 12(6), 350-354.

Copeland, D. R., deMoor, C., Moore, B. D., and Ater, J. L. (1999). Neurocognitive development of children after a cerebellar tumor in infancy: A longitudinal study. *Journal of Clinical Oncology*, 17(11), 3476-3486.

Daniels, C., Witt, K., Wolff, S., Jansen, O., and Deuschl, G. (2003). Rate dependency of the human cortical network subserving executive functions during generation of random number series: A functional magnetic resonance imaging study. *Neuroscience Letters*, 345(1), 25-28.

De Smet, H. J., Baillieux, H., Wackenier, P., De Praeter, M., Engelborghs, S., Paquier, P. F., De Deyn, P.P., and Marien, P. (2009). Long-term cognitive deficits following posterior fossa tumor resection: A neuropsychological and functional neuroimaging follow-up study. *Neuropsychology*, 23(6), 694-704.

Demirtas-Tatlidede, A., Freitas, C., Cromer, J. R., Safar, L., Ongur, D., Stone, W. S., ... and Pascual-Leone, A. (2010). Safety and proof of principle study of cerebellar vermal theta burst stimulation in refractory schizophrenia. *Schizophrenia Research,* 124(1-3), 91-100.

Doya, K. (2000). Complementary roles of basal ganglia and cerebellum in learning and motor control. *Current Opinion in Neurobiology*, 10(6), 732-739.

Dreher, J. C., and Grafman, J. (2002). The roles of the cerebellum and basal ganglia in timing and error prediction. *European Journal of Neuroscience*, 16(8), 1609-1619.

Durisko, C., and Fiez, J. A. (2010). Functional activation in the cerebellum during working memory and simple speech tasks. *Cortex*, 46(7), 896-906.

Ecker, C., Suckling, J., Deoni, S. C., Lombardo, M. V., Bullmore, E. T., Baron-Cohen, S., Catani, M., Jezzard, P., Barnes, A., Bailey, A.J., Williams, S.C., Murphy, D.G., and MRC AIMS Consortium (2012). Brain anatomy and its relationship to behavior in adults with autism spectrum disorder: A multicenter magnetic resonance imaging study. *Archives of General Psychiatry*, 69(2), 195-209.

Ernst, M., Bolla, K., Mouratidis, M., Contoreggi, C., Matochik, J. A., Kurian, V., Cadet, J.L., Kimes, A.S., and London, E. D. (2002). Decision-making in a risk-taking task: A PET study. *Neuropsychopharmacology*, 26(5), 682-691.

Exner, C., Weniger, G., and Irle, E. (2004). Cerebellar lesions in the PICA but not SCA territory impair cognition. *Neurology*, 63(11), 2132-2135.

Fatemi, S. H., Aldinger, K. A., Ashwood, P., Bauman, M. L., Blaha, C. D., Blatt, G. J., Chauhan, A., Chauhan, V., Dager, S.R., Dickson, P.E., Estes, A.M., Goldowitz, D., Heck, D.H., Kemper, T.L., King, B.H., Martin, L.A., Millen, K.J., Mittleman, G., Mosconi, M.W., Persico, A.M., Sweeney, J.A., Webb, S.J., and Welsh, J. P. (2012). Consensus paper: Pathological role of the cerebellum in autism. *Cerebellum*, 11(3), 777-807.

Fiez, J. A. and Raichle, M. E. (1997). Linguistic processing. *International Review of Neurobiology*, 41, 233-254.

Filippi, M., Canu, E., Gasparotti, R., Agosta, F., Valsecchi, P., Lodoli, G., Galluzzo, A., Comi, G., and Sacchetti, E. (2014). Patterns of brain structural changes in first-contact, antipsychotic drug-naive patients with schizophrenia. *American Journal of Neuroradiology*, 35(1), 30-37.

Fitzgerald, P. B., Laird, A. R., Maller, J., and Daskalakis, Z. J. (2008). A meta-analytic study of changes in brain activation in depression. *Human Brain Mapping*, 29(6), 683-695.

Frings, M., Dimitrova, A., Schorn, C. F., Elles, H. G., Hein-Kropp, C., Gizewski, E. R., Diener, H.C., and Timmann, D. (2006). Cerebellar involvement in verb generation: An fMRI study. *Neuroscience Letters*, 409(1), 19-23.

Fusar-Poli, P., Placentino, A., Carletti, F., Landi, P., Allen, P., Surguladze, S., Benedetti, F., Abbamonte, M., Gasparotti, R., Barale, F., Perez, J., McGuire, P., and Politi, P. (2009). Functional atlas of emotional faces processing: A voxel-based meta-analysis of 105 functional magnetic resonance imaging studies. *Journal of Psychiatry and Neuroscience*,34(6), 418-432.

Geday, J., Østergaard, K., Johnsen, E., and Gjedde, A. (2009). STN-stimulation in Parkinson's disease restores striatal inhibition of thalamocortical projection. *Human Brain Mapping*, 30(1), 112-121.

Gilbert, S. J., Bird, G., Brindley, R., Frith, C. D., and Burgess, P. W. (2008). Atypical recruitment of medial prefrontal cortex in autism spectrum disorders: An fMRI study of two executive function tasks. *Neuropsychologia,* 46(9), 2281-2291.

Gioia, G. A., Isquith, P. K., Guy, S. C., and Kenworthy, L. (2000). *BRIEF: Behavior Rating Inventory of Executive Function.* Lutz, Florida: Psychological Assessment Resources, Inc.

Gottwald, B., Wilde, B., Mihajlovic, Z., and Mehdorn, H. M. (2004). Evidence for distinct cognitive deficits after focal cerebellar lesions. *Journal of Neurology, Neurosurgery and Psychiatry*, 75(11), 1524-1531.

Grafman, J., Litvan, I., Massaquoi, S., Stewart, M., Sirigu, A., and Hallett, M. (1992). Cognitive planning deficit in patients with cerebellar atrophy. *Neurology,* 42(8), 1493-1496.

Grimaldi, G., Argyropoulos, G. P., Boehringer, A., Celnik, P., Edwards, M. J., Ferrucci, R., Galea, J.M., Groiss, S.J., Hiraoka, K., Kassavetis, P., Lesage, E., Manto, M., Miall, R.C., Priori, A., Sadnicka, A., Ugawa, Y., and Ziemann, U. (2014). Non-invasive cerebellar stimulation: A consensus paper. *Cerebellum,* 13(1), 121-138.

Grogan, A., Green, D. W., Ali, N., Crinion, J. T., and Price, C. J. (2009). Structural correlates of semantic and phonemic fluency ability in first and second languages. *Cerebral Cortex*, 19(11), 2690-2698.

Haines, D.E. (2014). Neuroanatomy in Clinical Context: An Atlas of Structures, Sections, Systems, and Syndromes. Philadelphia, PA: Wolters Kluwer Health.

Higuchi, S., Imamizu, H., and Kawato, M. (2007). Cerebellar activity evoked by common tool use execution and imagery tasks: An fMRI study. *Cortex,* 43(3), 350-358.

Hilker, R., Voges, J., Weisenbach, S., Kalbe, E., Burghaus, L., Ghaemi, M., Lehrke, R., Koulousakis, A., Herholz, K., Sturm, V., and Heiss, W. D. (2004). Subthalamic nucleus stimulation restores glucose metabolism in associative and limbic cortices and in cerebellum: Evidence from an FDG-PET study in advanced Parkinson's disease. *Journal of Cerebral Blood Flow and Metabolism,* 24(1), 7-16.

Hokkanen, L. S., Kauranen, V., Roine, R. O., Salonen, O., and Kotila, M. (2006). Subtle cognitive deficits after cerebellar infarcts. *European Journal of Neurology*, 13(2), 161-170.

Holmes, G. (1939). The cerebellum of man. *Brain*, 62(1), 1-30.

Hopyan, T., Laughlin, S., and Dennis, M. (2010). Emotions and their cognitive control in children with cerebellar tumors. *Journal of the International Neuropsychological Society*, 16(6), 1027-1038.

Hoshi, E., Tremblay, L., Féger, J., Carras, P. L., and Strick, P. L. (2005). The cerebellum communicates with the basal ganglia. *Nature Neuroscience*, 8(11), 1491-1493.

Huang, C., Mattis, P., Tang, C., Perrine, K., Carbon, M., and Eidelberg, D. (2007). Metabolic brain networks associated with cognitive function in Parkinson's disease. *Neuroimage*, 34(2), 714-723.

Ito, M. (1993). New concepts in cerebellar function. *Revue Neurologique*, 149(11), 596-599.

Ito, M. (2008). Control of mental activities by internal models in the cerebellum. *Nature Reviews: Neuroscience*, 9(4), 304-313.

Ito, M. (2010). *The Cerebellum: Brain for an Implicit Self*. Saddle River, NJ: Pearson Education.

Ito, M. (2013). Error detection and representation in the olivocerebellar system. *Frontiers in Neural Circuits*, 7, 1.

Jeong, J. W., Tiwari, V. N., Behen, M. E., Chugani, H. T., and Chugani, D. C. (2014). In vivo detection of reduced Purkinje cell fibers with diffusion MRI tractography in children with autistic spectrum disorders. *Frontiers in Human Neuroscience*, 8, 110.

Kalashnikova, L. A., Zueva, Y. V., Pugacheva, O. V., and Korsakova, N. K. (2005). Cognitive impairments in cerebellar infarcts. *Neuroscience and Behavioral Physiology*, 35(8), 773-779.

Karatekin, C., Lazareff, J. A., and Asarnow, R. F. (2000). Relevance of the cerebellar hemispheres for executive functions. *Pediatric Neurology*, 22(2), 106-112.

Kathmann, N., Rupertseder, C., Hauke, W., and Zaudig, M. (2005). Implicit sequence learning in obsessive-compulsive disorder: Further support for the fronto-striatal dysfunction model *Biological Psychiatry*, 58(3), 233-238.

Kenworthy, L., Yerys, B. E., Anthony, L. G., and Wallace, G. L. (2008). Understanding executive control in autism spectrum disorders in the lab and in the real world. *Neuropsychology Review*, 18(4), 320-338.

Khadka, S., Meda, S. A., Stevens, M. C., Glahn, D. C., Calhoun, V. D., Sweeney, J. A., Tamminga, C.A., Keshavan, M.S., O'Neil, K., Schretlen, D., and Pearlson, G. D. (2013). Is aberrant functional connectivity a psychosis endophenotype? A resting state functional magnetic resonance imaging study. *Bioligical Psychiatry*, 74(6), 458-466.

Koch, G. (2010). Repetitive transcranial magnetic stimulation: A tool for human cerebellar plasticity. *Functional Neurology*, 25(3), 159-163.

Koch, K., Wagner, G., Dahnke, R., Schachtzabel, C., Schultz, C., Roebel, M., Güllmar, D., Reichenbach, J.R., Sauer, H., and Schlosser, R. G. (2010). Disrupted white matter integrity of corticopontine-cerebellar circuitry in schizophrenia. *European Archives of Psychiatry and Clinical Neuroscience,* 260(5), 419-426.

Koziol, L. F., and Budding, D. E. (2009). *Subcortical Structures and Cognition: Implications for Neuropsychological Assessment.* New York, NY: Springer.

Koziol, L. F., Budding, D. E., and Chidekel, D. (2012). From movement to thought: executive function, embodied cognition, and the cerebellum. *The Cerebellum*, 11(2), 505-525.

Krain, A. L., and Castellanos, F. X. (2006). Brain development and ADHD. *Clinical Psychology Review*, 26(4), 433-444.

Krienen, F. M., and Buckner, R. L. (2009). Segregated frontocerebellar circuits revealed by intrinsic functional connectivity. *Cerebral Cortex,* 19(10), 2485-2497.

Kuhn, S., Romanowski, A., Schubert, F., and Gallinat, J. (2012). Reduction of cerebellar grey matter in Crus I and II in schizophrenia. *Brain Structure and Function,* 217(2), 523-529.

Lerner, A., Bagic, A., Boudreau, E. A., Hanakawa, T., Pagan, F., Mari, Z., Bara-Jimenez, W., Aksu, M., Garraux, G., Simmons, J.M., Sato, S., Murphy, D.L., and Hallett, M. (2007). Neuroimaging of neuronal circuits involved in tic generation in patients with Tourette syndrome. *Neurology,* 68(23), 1979-1987.

Levisohn, L., Cronin-Golomb, A., and Schmahmann, J. D. (2000). Neuropsychological consequences of cerebellar tumour resection in children: Cerebellar cognitive affective syndrome in a paediatric population. *Brain,* 123 (Pt 5), 1041-1050.

Lie, C. H., Specht, K., Marshall, J. C., and Fink, G. R. (2006). Using fMRI to decompose the neural processes underlying the Wisconsin Card Sorting Test. *Neuroimage,* 30(3), 1038-1049.

Lungu, O., Barakat, M., Laventure, S., Debas, K., Proulx, S., Luck, D., and Stip, E. (2013). The incidence and nature of cerebellar findings in schizophrenia: A quantitative review of fMRI literature. *Schizophrrenia Bulletin,* 39(4), 797-806.

Luna, B., Doll, S. K., Hegedus, S. J., Minshew, N. J., and Sweeney, J. A. (2007). Maturation of executive function in autism. *Biological Psychiatry*, 61(4), 474-481.

Luna, B., Minshew, N. J., Garver, K. E., Lazar, N. A., Thulborn, K. R., Eddy, W. F., and Sweeney, J. A. (2002). Neocortical system abnormalities in autism: An fMRI study of spatial working memory. *Neurology*, 59(6), 834-840.

Makris, N., Liang, L., Biederman, J., Valera, E. M., Brown, A. B., Petty, C., Spencer, T.J., Faraone, S.V., and Seidman, L. J. (in press). Toward defining the neural substrates of ADHD: A controlled structural MRI study in medication-naive adults. *Journal of Attention Disorders.*

Manes, F., Villamil, A. R., Ameriso, S., Roca, M., and Torralva, T. (2009). "Real life" executive deficits in patients with focal vascular lesions affecting the cerebellum. *Journal of Neurological Sciences*, 283(1-2), 95-98.

Marien, P., Baillieux, H., De Smet, H. J., Engelborghs, S., Wilssens, I., Paquier, P., and De Deyn, P. P. (2009). Cognitive, linguistic and affective disturbances following a right superior cerebellar artery infarction: A case study. *Cortex,* 45(4), 527-536.

Marvel, C. L., and Desmond, J. E. (2010). Functional topography of the cerebellum in verbal working memory. *Neuropsychology Review*, 20(3), 271-279.

Massat, I., Slama, H., Kavec, M., Linotte, S., Mary, A., Baleriaux, D., Metens, T., Mendlewicz, J., and Peigneux, P. (2012). Working memory-related functional brain patterns in never medicated children with ADHD. *PLoS ONE,* 7(11), e49392.

McAlonan, G. M., Cheung, V., Chua, S. E., Oosterlaan, J., Hung, S. F., Tang, C. P., Lee, C.C., Kwong, S.L., Ho, T.P., Cheung, C., Suckling, J., and Leung, P. W. (2009). Age-related grey matter volume correlates of response inhibition and shifting in attention-deficit hyperactivity disorder. *British Joutrnal of Psychiatry*, 194(2), 123-129.

Menzies, L., Chamberlain, S. R., Laird, A. R., Thelen, S. M., Sahakian, B. J., and Bullmore, E. T. (2008). Integrating evidence from neuroimaging and neuropsychological studies of obsessive-compulsive disorder: the orbitofronto-striatal model revisited. *Neuroscience and Biobehavioral Reviews,* 32(3), 525-549.

Mostofsky, S. H., Reiss, A. L., Lockhart, P., and Denckla, M. B. (1998). Evaluation of cerebellar size in attention-deficit hyperactivity disorder. *Journal of Child Neurology*, 13 (9), 434-439.

Meyer-Lindenberg, A. S., Olsen, R. K., Kohn, P. D., Brown, T., Egan, M. F., Weinberger, D. R., and Berman, K. F. (2005). Regionally specific disturbance of dorsolateral prefrontal-hippocampal functional connectivity in schizophrenia. *Archives of General Psychiatry*, 62(4), 379-386.

Nagahama, Y., Fukuyama, H., Yamauchi, H., Matsuzaki, S., Konishi, J., Shibasaki, H., and Kimura, J. (1996). Cerebral activation during performance of a card sorting test. *Brain,* 119 (Pt 5), 1667-1675.

Parvizi, J., Anderson, S. W., Martin, C. O., Damasio, H., and Damasio, A. R. (2001). Pathological laughter and crying: A link to the cerebellum. *Brain,* 124(Pt 9), 1708-1719.

Parvizi, J., Joseph, J., Press, D. Z., and Schmahmann, J. D. (2007). Pathological laughter and crying in patients with multiple system atrophy-cerebellar type. *Movement Disorders,* 22 (6), 798-803.

Peng, J., Liu, J., Nie, B., Li, Y., Shan, B., Wang, G., and Li, K. (2011). Cerebral and cerebellar gray matter reduction in first-episode patients with major depressive disorder: A voxel-based morphometry study. *European Journal of Radiology,* 80(2), 395-399.

Picard, H., Amado, I., Mouchet-Mages, S., Olie, J. P., and Krebs, M. O. (2008). The role of the cerebellum in schizophrenia: An update of clinical, cognitive, and functional evidences. *Schizophrenia Bulletin*, 34(1), 155-172.

Pillay, S. S., Yurgelun-Todd, D. A., Bonello, C. M., Lafer, B., Fava, M., and Renshaw, P. F. (1997). A quantitative magnetic resonance imaging study of cerebral and cerebellar gray matter volume in primary unipolar major depression: Relationship to treatment response and clinical severity. *Biological Psychiatry*, 42(2), 79-84.

Qiu, J., Li, H., Jou, J., Liu, J., Luo, Y., Feng, T., Wu, Z., and Zhang, Q. (2010). Neural correlates of the "Aha" experiences: evidence from an fMRI study of insight problem solving. *Cortex*, 46(3), 397-403.

Ramnani, N., Behrens, T. E., Johansen-Berg, H., Richter, M. C., Pinsk, M. A., Andersson, J. L., Rudebeck, P., Ciccarelli, O., Richter, W., Thompson, A.J., Gross, C.G., Robson, M.D., Kastner, S., and Matthews, P. M. (2006). The evolution of prefrontal inputs to the cortico-pontine system: Diffusion imaging evidence from macaque monkeys and humans. *Cerebral Cortex*, 16(6), 811-818.

Rasser, P. E., Schall, U., Peck, G., Cohen, M., Johnston, P., Khoo, K., Carr, V.J., Ward, P.B., Thompson, P. M. (2010). Cerebellar grey matter deficits in first-episode schizophrenia mapped using cortical pattern matching. *Neuroimage,* 53(4), 1175-1180.

Rapin, L., Poissant, H., and Mendrek, A. (in press). Atypical activations of frontocerebellar regions during forethought in parents of children with ADHD. *Journal of Attention Disorders.*

Ravizza, S. M., and Ivry, R. B. (2001). Comparison of the basal ganglia and cerebellum in shifting attention. *Journal of Cognitive Neuroscience*, 13(3), 285-297.

Richter, S., Gerwig, M., Aslan, B., Wilhelm, H., Schoch, B., Dimitrova, A., Gizewski, E.R., Ziegler, W., Karnath, H.O., and Timmann, D. (2007). Cognitive functions in patients with MR defined chronic focal cerebellar lesions. *Journal of Neurology,* 254(9), 1193-1203.

Ropper, A. H., and Samuels, M. A. (2009). *Adams and Victor's Principles of Neurology,* 9th Ed. New York, NY: McGraw Hill Medical.

Rosenthal, M., Wallace, G. L., Lawson, R., Wills, M. C., Dixon, E., Yerys, B. E., and Kenworthy, L. (2013). Impairments in real world executive function increase from childhood to adolescence in autism spectrum disorders. *Neuropsychology,* 27(1), 13-18.

Roth, R. M., Baribeau, J., Milovan, D., O'Connor, K., and Todorov, C. (2004). Procedural and declarative memory in obsessive-compulsive disorder. *Journal of the International Neuropsychological Society*, 10(5), 647-654.

Roth, R. M., Lavoie, M., Mason, E. A., and O'Connor, K. (2013). Obsessive-compulsive disorder. In C. A. Noggle and R. S. Dean (Eds.), *The Neuropsychological of Psychopathology*, (pp. 261-286). New York, NY: Springer Publishing Company.

Roth, R. M., and Saykin, A. J. (2004). Executive dysfunction in attention-deficit/hyperactivity disorder: Cognitive and neuroimaging findings. *Psychiatric Clinics of North America*, 27(1), 83-96.

Roth, R. M., Saykin, A. J., Flashman, L. A., Pixley, H. S., West, J. D., and Mamourian, A. C. (2007). Event-related functional magnetic resonance imaging of response inhibition in obsessive-compulsive disorder. *Biological psychiatry*, 62(8), 901-909.

Schall, U., Johnston, P., Lagopoulos, J., Juptner, M., Jentzen, W., Thienel, R., Dittmann-Balçar, A., Bender, S., and Ward, P. B. (2003). Functional brain maps of Tower of London performance: A positron emission tomography and functional magnetic resonance imaging study. *Neuroimage*, 20(2), 1154-1161.

Schienle, A., and Scharmuller, W. (2013). Cerebellar activity and connectivity during the experience of disgust and happiness. *Neuroscience*, 246, 375-381.

Schlosser, R., Gesierich, T., Kaufmann, B., Vucurevic, G., Hunsche, S., Gawehn, J., and Stoeter, P. (2003). Altered effective connectivity during working memory performance in schizophrenia: A study with fMRI and structural equation modeling. *Neuroimage*, 19(3), 751-763.

Schmahmann, J. D. (1998). Dysmetria of thought: Clinical consequences of cerebellar dysfunction on cognition and affect. *Trends in Cognitive Sciences,* 2(9), 362-371.

Schmahmann, J. D. (2000). The role of the cerebellum in affect and psychosis. *Journal of Neurolinguistics*, 13(2), 189-214.

Schmahmann, J. D., and Pandya, D. N. (1997). The cerebrocerebellar system. *International Review of Neurobiology*, 41, 31-60.

Schmahmann, J. D., and Sherman, J. C. (1998). The cerebellar cognitive affective syndrome. *Brain*, 121(4), 561-579.

Schmahmann, J. D., Weilburg, J. B., and Sherman, J. C. (2007). The neuropsychiatry of the cerebellum: Insights from the clinic. *Cerebellum,* 6(3), 254-267.

Schmitz, C., and Rezaie, P. (2008). The neuropathology of autism: where do we stand? *Neuropathology and Applied Neurobiology*, 34(1), 4-11.

Schutter, D. J., Enter, D., and Hoppenbrouwers, S. S. (2009). High-frequency repetitive transcranial magnetic stimulation to the cerebellum and implicit processing of happy facial expressions. *Journal of Psychiatry and Neuroscience,* 34(1), 60-65.

Schutter, D. J., and van Honk, J. (2009). The cerebellum in emotion regulation: A repetitive transcranial magnetic stimulation study. *Cerebellum,* 8(1), 28-34.

Schutter, D. J., van Honk, J., d'Alfonso, A. A., Peper, J. S., and Panksepp, J. (2003). High frequency repetitive transcranial magnetic over the medial cerebellum induces a shift in the prefrontal electroencephalography gamma spectrum: A pilot study in humans. *Neuroscience Letters*, 336(2), 73-76.

Schweizer, T. A., Alexander, M. P., Susan Gillingham, B. A., Cusimano, M., and Stuss, D. T. (2010). Lateralized cerebellar contributions to word generation: A phonemic and semantic fluency study. *Behavioral Neurology,* 23(1-2), 31-37.

Schweizer, T. A., Levine, B., Rewilak, D., O'Connor, C., Turner, G., Alexander, M. P., Cusimano, M., Manly, T., Robertson, I.H., and Stuss, D. T. (2008). Rehabilitation of executive functioning after focal damage to the cerebellum. *Neurorehabilitation and Neural Repair*, 22(1), 72-77.

Scott, J. A., Schumann, C. M., Goodlin-Jones, B. L., and Amaral, D. G. (2009). A comprehensive volumetric analysis of the cerebellum in children and adolescents with autism spectrum disorder. *Autism Research*, 2(5), 246-257.

Seidman, L. J., Valera, E. M., and Makris, N. (2005). Structural brain imaging of attention-deficit/hyperactivity disorder. *Biological Psychiatry*, 57(11), 1263-1272.

Segarra, N., Bernardo, M., Valdes, M., Caldu, X., Falcon, C., Rami, L., Bargallo, N., Parramon, G., and Junque, C. (2008). Cerebellar deficits in schizophrenia are associated with executive dysfunction. *NeuroReport,* 19(15), 1513-1517.

Seo, D., Olman, C. A., Haut, K. M., Sinha, R., Macdonald, A. W., and Patrick, C. J. (2014). Neural correlates of preparatory and regulatory control over positive and negative emotion. *Social, Cognitive and Affective Neuroscience,* 9(4), 494-504.

Shah, S. A., Doraiswamy, P. M., Husain, M. M., Escalona, P. R., Na, C., Figiel, G. S., Patterson, L.J., Ellinwood, E.H. Jr, McDonald, W.M., and Krishnan, K.R. (1992). Posterior fossa abnormalities in major depression: A controlled magnetic resonance imaging study. *Acta Psychiatrica Scandinavica,* 85(6), 474-479.

Singer, T., Seymour, B., O'Doherty, J., Kaube, H., Dolan, R. J., and Frith, C. D. (2004). Empathy for pain involves the affective but not sensory components of pain. *Science,* 303 (5661), 1157-1162.

Sivaswamy, L., Kumar, A., Rajan, D., Behen, M., Muzik, O., Chugani, D., and Chugani, H. (2010). A diffusion tensor imaging study of the cerebellar pathways in children with autism spectrum disorder. *Journal of Child Neurology,* 25(10), 1223-1231.

Snyder, H. R. (2013). Major depressive disorder is associated with broad impairments on neuropsychological measures of executive function: A meta-analysis and review. *Psychological Bulletin*, 139(1), 81-132.

Speer, A. M., Kimbrell, T. A., Wassermann, E. M., J, D. R., Willis, M. W., Herscovitch, P., and Post, R. M. (2000). Opposite effects of high and low frequency rTMS on regional brain activity in depressed patients. *Biological Psychiatry*, 48(12), 1133-1141.

Stoodley, C. J., and Schmahmann, J. D. (2009). Functional topography in the human cerebellum: A meta-analysis of neuroimaging studies. *Neuroimage*, 44(2), 489-501.

Stuss, D. T., and Alexander, M. P. (2000). Executive functions and the frontal lobes: A conceptual view. *Psychological Research*, 63(3-4), 289-298.

Su, T. W., Lan, T. H., Hsu, T. W., Biswal, B. B., Tsai, P. J., Lin, W. C., and Lin, C. P. (2013). Reduced neuro-integration from the dorsolateral prefrontal cortex to the whole brain and executive dysfunction in schizophrenia patients and their relatives. *Schizophrenia Research*, 148(1-3), 50-58.

Tamm, L., and Juranek, J. (2012). Fluid reasoning deficits in children with ADHD: Evidence from fMRI. *Brain Research*, 1465, 48-56.

Tobe, R. H., Bansal, R., Xu, D., Hao, X., Liu, J., Sanchez, J., and Peterson, B. S. (2010). Cerebellar morphology in Tourette syndrome and obsessive-compulsive disorder. *Annals of Neurology*, 67(4), 479-487.

Torriero, S., Oliveri, M., Koch, G., Lo Gerfo, E., Salerno, S., Petrosini, L., and Caltagirone, C. (2007). Cortical networks of procedural learning: Evidence from cerebellar damage. Neuropsychologia, 45(6), 1208-1214.

Turner, B. M., Paradiso, S., Marvel, C. L., Pierson, R., Boles Ponto, L. L., Hichwa, R. D., and Robinson, R. G. (2007). The cerebellum and emotional experience. *Neuropsychologia,* 45 (6), 1331-1341.

Valera, E. M., Faraone, S. V., Biederman, J., Poldrack, R. A., and Seidman, L. J. (2005). Functional neuroanatomy of working memory in adults with attention-deficit/ hyperactivity disorder. *Biological Psychiatry*, 57(5), 439-447.

Vaquero, E., Gomez, C. M., Quintero, E. A., Gonzalez-Rosa, J. J., and Marquez, J. (2008). Differential prefrontal-like deficit in children after cerebellar astrocytoma and medulloblastoma tumor. *Behavior and Brain Function,* 4, 18.

Vasic, N., Walter, H., Sambataro, F., and Wolf, R. C. (2009). Aberrant functional connectivity of dorsolateral prefrontal and cingulate networks in patients with major depression during working memory processing. *Psychological Medicine*, 39(6), 977-987.

Vloet, T. D., Gilsbach, S., Neufang, S., Fink, G. R., Herpertz-Dahlmann, B., and Konrad, K. (2010). Neural mechanisms of interference control and time discrimination in attention-deficit/hyperactivity disorder. *Journal of the American Academy of Child and Adolescent Psychiatry,* 49(4), 356-367.

Wang, S., Yang, Y., Xing, W., Chen, J., Liu, C., and Luo, X. (2013). Altered neural circuits related to sustained attention and executive control in children with ADHD: An event-related fMRI study. *Clinical Neurophysiology*, 124(11), 2181-2190.

Watson, D. R., Anderson, J. M., Bai, F., Barrett, S. L., McGinnity, T. M., Mulholland, C. C., Rushe, T.M., Cooper, S. J. (2012). A voxel based morphometry study investigating brain structural changes in first episode psychosis. *Behavioural Brain Research*, 227(1), 91-99.

White, T., Schmidt, M., Kim, D. I., and Calhoun, V. D. (2011). Disrupted functional brain connectivity during verbal working memory in children and adolescents with schizophrenia. *Cerebral Cortex*, 21(3), 510-518.

Wolf, R. C., Plichta, M. M., Sambataro, F., Fallgatter, A. J., Jacob, C., Lesch, K. P., Herrmann, M.J., Schönfeldt-Lecuona, C., Connemann, B.J., Grön, G., and Vasic, N. (2009). Regional brain activation changes and abnormal functional connectivity of the ventrolateral prefrontal cortex during working memory processing in adults with attention-deficit/hyperactivity disorder. *Human Brain Mapping*, 30(7), 2252-2266.

Yang, Y., Kim, J. E., Lee, J. S., and Kim, S. (2007). Akinetic mutism and cognitive affective syndrome caused by unilateral pica infarction. *Journal of Clinical Neurology*, 3(4), 192-196.

Yucel, K., Nazarov, A., Taylor, V. H., Macdonald, K., Hall, G. B., and Macqueen, G. M. (2013). Cerebellar vermis volume in major depressive disorder. *Brain Structure and Function*, 218(4), 851-858.

Ziemus, B., Baumann, O., Luerding, R., Schlosser, R., Schuierer, G., Bogdahn, U., and Greenlee, M. W. (2007). Impaired working memory after cerebellar infarcts paralleled by changes in BOLD signal of a corticocerebellar circuit. *Neuropsychologia,* 45(9), 2016-2024.

Zoccatelli, G., Beltramello, A., Alessandrini, F., Pizzini, F. B., and Tassinari, G. (2010). Word and position interference in stroop tasks: A behavioral and fMRI study. *Experimental Brain Research*, 207(1-2), 139-147.

INDEX

A

B

C

D

E

F

G

H

I

L

M

Q

R

S

T

U

V

W

Y